"As a clinician and practicir Brunk's journey to health a m suffers with debilitating illnes. *Diseases and Me* is an inspiring, informative and upinimg book. Ron points the direction to wholeness, gives the reader insight, and holds your hand all along the way. It's a gem of an opportunity for today's overburdened and over-consuming lifestyle practitioners."

– Dena Bazzie
LPC, LMFT, NBCC, CTS, CEAP

"This book is a captivating account of a man's personal journey through spiritual, mental, emotional and physical despair. The clarity and openness with which Ron Brunk describes his journey was enlightening for me, providing a glimpse into the terrifying world of a person who has been living with mysterious diseases for many years. For healthcare practitioners of all kinds, in both conventional and complementary medicine, this book delivers a patient perspective that speaks to the heart and reminds us that patients are persons, not just diseases."

"Equally, I'm sure, for those persons who are struggling with their own mysterious diseases, many will resonate with aspects of Ron Brunk's story. He has found peace through acceptance of his own humanity, but in doing so has become a testament to the wonder of human resilience. His very easy to read and frank advice has the potential to change lives."

– Kate Chatfield MSc FHEA
Course Leader MSc Integrated Healthcare
School of Health
University of Central Lancashire
Preston, England

"Ron Brunk's *Mystery Diseases and Me* is spot on. It articulates a truth about the daunting struggle that many of my clients face. This struggle can be overwhelming and bewildering at times. Stress-related illnesses, mystery illnesses, are the result of forces that seem beyond their control. Often folks feel completely helpless in the face of these problems, and on top of that are often made to feel 'crazy' by the medical establishment. Ron's book will provide hope, humor and meaning to the struggle to gain control over one's own life. Each one of my clients could use a copy!"

– Edward L. Brinson, LCSW
www.parenttopics.blogspot.com

"Ron Brunk shares his awesome story with humor, candor and his unique take on love, faith, healing & hope. It is a heartwarming story of one man's journey to joy through amazing trials and tribulations of mind, body and spirit. Brunk emerges triumphant with a wonderful message of perseverance for all who have suffered. *Mystery Diseases & Me* succeeds as a life-affirming, honest to God adventure! It's a modern day fable."

– Billy Block, Producer/Host/Musician
Life-Long Positivist and Serial Meditator
www.billyblock.com

"Ron Brunk's candid story of incredible physical and emotional challenge has brought forth a message of great spiritual wisdom for a suffering world."

– Reverend Dr. Linda Marie Nelson, OSR
Instructor at Metropolitan Theological Seminary

"*Mystery Diseases and Me* is Ron Brunk's tale of health horrors, decline, and then recovery. He finds the wisdom to understand that life is about <u>Balance</u> and the <u>Choices</u> we make. In order to be healthy, your health must be a priority, and Ron gets it. Good nutrition, exercise, sleep, and a support network are the cornerstones, while 'de-stressing' the core provides a strong framework to build upon. If all my patients would work on constructing a healthy mind and body then some might be cured of their 'mystery disease,' but all would be better in the long run."

– Tad Yoneyama, M.D.
Vanderbilt Medical Center

[Dr. Tad Yoneyama is board certified in Internal Medicine and Pediatrics, a clinical faculty member of Vanderbilt Medical Center, a former varsity athlete at Duke University, and an organic gardener. Dr. Yoneyama has patients living across the United States from California to New York, in Europe, and also in Asia who still come back to see him regularly.]

"Ron Brunk's book relates his frightening story in an entertaining manner, and demonstrates how he moved from victim to victor over his mystery diseases. A great read for anyone facing health challenges."

– Laura Duksta
New York Times* bestselling author, *I Love You More
***(aka* The Bald Chick due to the auto-immune**
condition Alopecia Areata)

"Medicine, especially family medicine, is a humbling business. I stress to my patients that there is often not a right answer; we just do the best we can to work together to find a solution. Ron Brunk accurately portrays in his book that there are many mystery diseases which are hard to diagnose and difficult to treat."

"My mentor, the renowned Dr. John Hendrick, often told me, 'Always listen to your patients; they will tell you what is wrong with them. And if you listen long enough, they will help you understand how to fix them.' Sometimes just listening to a patient does more good than any pill I can give them."

"I urge you to read *Mystery Diseases and Me*; it will help you to 'Ask not what life can do for me, but what can I do for life?' Congratulations to Ron Brunk for writing this inspiring book that will aid other patients and physicians too."

– Kelly M. Pitsenbarger, M.D.

[Dr. Kelly M. Pitsenbarger has been in practice for 27 years, and has been a member of the WVAFP (West Virginia Academy of Family Practice) Legislative Committee since 2000. He served as WVAFP President in 2004-2005, and as WVAFP Secretary in 2001. Dr. Pitsenbarger has been a fellow for the AAFP since 2004, and also serves as a WV Alternate Delegate.]

"Ron Brunk is a friend of mine, the newest old friend that I have. We felt like old friends the first time that I met him as a keyboardist/vocalist on one of his recording sessions. Ironically, the name of the track (and one of my favorites of his) is a song called 'Vitamin Me'. We hit it off instantly."

"As a musician and a closet nutritionist I really enjoyed this story of Ron's journey, and find it fascinating that a book that offers me little in nutritional answers offers me so much in what it takes to make it through life happy, whole, and inspired. I loved it. I read it in one sitting, and I *never* do that."

"Every time I see Ron, we pick up where we left off before and talk for hours. After reading this account of his life, I am sure we have another long, enriching conversation ahead."

**– Joseph A. Wooten, Hands of Soul
Keyboardist/Vocalist for the Steve Miller Band**

"One remarkable man's journey through the long nightmare of our dis-ease and disease-focused world of modern human distress; a journey that often initially manifests with simple, yet overwhelming anxiety, as it did with Ron. As his mystery diseases manifested, so did his despair, but as many of us are now starting to learn: we enter this journey feeling utterly broken and terrified, and yet if we have the courage to reach in all directions for ultimate truth and meaning, we discover that the journey itself can bring the realization that we, in time, find ourselves on the cutting edge of human possibility. Thank you Ron, for inspiring anyone who will have a look here."

**– Bedford M. Combs, LMFT, Founder of Heartstream
Journeys Personal Growth and Training Programs**

"Based on my 38 years of hands-on patient care as a licensed practical nurse, I believe that Ron Brunk's book is a must-read for anyone who wants to be more in tune with their own body."

– Debra Ewing, LPN

"Mystery Diseases and Me" is a very compelling read. The book is a journey of the human spirit through the words of a man whose life has been a roller coaster of emotion, pain, extreme trials and finally perseverance. As a licensed social worker I highly recommend this book to those who are hurting."

– Michael S. Horton, MSW, LSW

"Ron Brunk's tale is an enlightening exposé of personal struggle; offering both help and a path of hope."

– William Beck
author of the Bryson McGann novels
www.booksbybeck.com

"Ron Brunk is not only an immensely talented singer-songwriter, he's also an open book allowing himself to become vulnerable about his journey in the hope of helping others. This book in its honesty will encourage any and everyone who has ever been nagged with the thought that 'something is wrong – why can't anyone help me?'"

– Devon O'Day
Author-Speaker-Personality Mix 92.9/ Nashville

"Ron has a marvelous, easy to read writing style that is quite rare. This is not a diagnostic textbook; instead, the author shares his real life experiences of adversity and does a great job of taking the reader along on his journey."

– Charlie Yeargan, Ph.D.,
Licensed Clinical Psychologist

"Mr. Brunk hits the nail on the head in this book. As a medical provider with over 20 years in practice, I have also been a patient with similar experiences and health challenges. This very thing inspired me to help those with 'Mystery Diseases' in my clinical practice. Mr. Brunk's book brings a heightened and much needed awareness to both the medical community and the health care consumer. It often seems as though common sense is put on the back burner, and patients are treated according to numbers on a piece of paper; but there is much more to a human being than their lab results."

"We have done an excellent job in our sick-care system of segregating patients into 'pieces;' however, the hip bone really is connected to the knee bone, just as the thyroid is really connected to the adrenal glands and hypothalamus. Only by marrying conventional and 'WHOLE-istic' medicine can we achieve a win-win situation."

"This book tells the story of one man's amazing transition from frustration, hopelessness, and desperation to encouragement, self-awareness, intuition and motivation. It is a testimony to the multitude of patients who continue to have unanswered questions and find themselves living in their own dark abyss."

– Paige Adams, FNP, B-C, MAPS
Fellow Owner, The Center for Proactive Medicine

For Tracie.

For Ashley, Meagan, and Michael.

I owe so much to so many, and offer up my deepest
gratitude to each and every one who has ever loved,
supported, and believed in me.
Thank you for your kindness and generosity.
You have my forever love.
May goodness be showered upon you.

MYSTERY DISEASES AND ME

My Battle With

Fibromyalgia
Intestinal Hemorrhaging
Obsessive Compulsive Disorder
Eating Disorders
Irritable Bowel Syndrome
Bipolar Disorder
Anxiety Disorders ▪ Panic Attacks
Manic Depressive Disorder
Adrenal Fatigue ▪ Anemia
Depression ▪ Shingles
Chronic Fatigue & Chronic Pain Syndromes
Alcoholism ▪ Agoraphobia
Post-Traumatic Stress Disorder
Connective Tissue Disease
Retinal Vein Occlusion ▪ Tinnitus
Degenerative Arthritis
Restless Leg Syndrome ▪ Spinal Stenosis
Diverticulosis ▪ Benign Fasciculation Syndrome
Lactose Intolerance ▪ Gluten Sensitivity
Chronic Prostatitis
and
Modern Medicine

By RON BRUNK

Printed in the United States of America

ISBN 978-0-989737-20-3 (eBook)
ISBN 978-0-9897372-1-0 (pbk)

Library of Congress Control Number 2013945509

Cover design by Tracy Lucas of Four Square Creative.

Alexia Publishing
PO Box 120942
Nashville, TN 37212

www.AlexiaPublishing.com

www.MysteryDiseasesAndMe.com

www.RonBrunk.com

ronbrunk@comcast.net

Contents

MYSTERY DISEASES AND ME

A Note from the Author

Dear Reader:

For nearly twenty years I have waged a very personal and desperate battle for my own life. I have endured three separate attacks of massive, life-threatening, intestinal hemorrhages that required transfusions to save me. I have also been diagnosed along the way with nearly thirty painful diseases, disorders, and syndromes including fibromyalgia, agoraphobia, irritable bowel syndrome, numerous anxiety disorders, depression, post-traumatic stress disorder, panic attacks, manic-depressive disorder, chronic prostatitis, adrenal fatigue, anemia, and obsessive-compulsive disorder.

This book tells the story of my journey. It describes some of my manic-depressive behaviors, near-death experiences, trials and tribulations with doctors and drugs, terrifying panic attacks, and suicidal moments. Most importantly, *Mystery Diseases and Me* describes the spiritual and life lessons I learned along the way. I hope that this book will encourage, inform, and aid you as you unravel the secrets of your own mystery diseases, and discover the beautiful path to healing.

Love and peace,
Ron Brunk
August 28, 2013

Mystery Diseases and Me

Preface

The Merriam-Webster Dictionary defines the word "disease" as *a condition of the living animal or plant body or one of its parts that impairs normal functioning and is typically manifested by distinguishing signs and symptoms: sickness, malady.*

I coined the expression "mystery disease" for the purposes of this book; and intentionally use the term "disease" in the broadest sense of the word, as a catch-all description for any poorly understood ailment (with or without an apparent organic cause) that afflicts the human being. Of course, applying a label to anything – particularly an illness, disease, or syndrome – can be a challenging task, fraught with second-guessing and differing opinions.

I am aware that, medically speaking, there may be a variety of technical distinctions between the following words: disease, disorder, functional disorder, illness, ailment, syndrome, condition, and sickness. But for the sake of layman's simplicity and the intents of this book, I will often use these terms interchangeably; grouping them all under the generalized, umbrella expression "mystery diseases."

Few, if any, diseases or disorders are fully and completely understood by medical science. Most still retain a varying degree of mystery regarding their origin, method of transmission, prevalence, prevention, treatment strategies, or cure. Some illnesses, such as fibromyalgia or Alzheimer's, remain mostly shrouded in mystery, and few would argue that they can be appropriately labeled as "mystery diseases."

Others maladies, however, may not be as easily defined and categorized. For some of them, medical science has discovered an organic cause – Crohn's disease, for example – but still has little idea how to effectively treat or cure it. While in other cases such as diabetes or asthma, effective treatment regimens have been determined, but the cause or other aspects of the diseases remain somewhat of an enigma.

Therefore, I have taken the liberty of assigning the "mystery" description to particular illnesses described in this book, based on my own subjective assessment of the full scope of man's understanding of each ailment. From Parkinson's disease to Pica Disorder, from Farmer's Lung to Q Fever, and from Burning Feet Syndrome to Watermelon Stomach, there is a world of mystery diseases out there waiting for us to solve.

The Bad News

Mystery diseases rarely show up on blood work, CAT scans, MRI, ultrasound, or any other type of conventional test or exam. They are the disorders of unknown origin that your doctor must diagnose primarily by process of elimination. Mystery diseases are the illnesses that medical science does not yet understand or know how to effectively treat. And worst of all, they're the afflictions that bring daily misery to at least one hundred million Americans, nearly a third of the population of the United States.

As shown in Chart A, 40 million American citizens suffer from anxiety disorders, 23.8 million have a mood disorder such as depression, at least six million battle fibromyalgia, and as many as 45 million suffer from some form of Irritable Bowel Syndrome (IBS) or other gastrointestinal disease.

Even the most casual observer cannot deny that there seems to be a rising tide of mystery diseases plaguing our society, and causing multitudes to suffer a disturbing array of neurological, gastrointestinal, mood, musculoskeletal, bleeding, and autoimmune disorders.

Sadly, there are far too many examples of mystery diseases all around me, as many of my family and friends are victims of these insidious disorders. Two suffer with debilitating migraines for which no cause or remedy can be found. Another endures the fiery agony of erythromelalgia, the "burning feet" syndrome, and is forced to soak her feet in buckets of ice water at least a dozen times a day to lessen the pain. As with most of the mystery diseases, doctors have absolutely no idea what causes this malady or how to treat it.

Crohn's disease recently claimed the life of one of my friends, and several others also suffer the ongoing misery and embarrassment of this or other gastrointestinal problems. Huntington's disease claimed one of my relatives, and depression led to the death of a close friend. Many more are battling the unending pain of fibromyalgia and the terror of anxiety disorders and panic attacks.

Finally, one young man who is very close to me has been stricken by a slew of mysterious and debilitating symptoms. A few months ago he was a strong, vibrant member of the United States Air Force, a world traveler who had been to every continent on the planet. Now, as a result of the onslaught of several mystery diseases, he is nearly incapacitated and facing a medical discharge from the job and military service he loves so dearly. His team of doctors remains dumbfounded.

I am aware that there are people who believe that I am making much ado about nothing. Some think that these mysterious ailments are simply the complaints of weak-willed people and hypochondriacs. Having never personally experienced the pain and misery of a mystery disease, the naysayers are skeptical of our symptoms and complaints. *It's all in your head*, they say.

I confess I once shared that view, until life taught me a very tough lesson. This book is the story of my schooling – what I lived and what I learned as a result.

Chart A: MYSTERY DISEASES IN THE U.S.

DISEASE/DISORDER (est. cases in millions)		Source*
Irritable Bowel Syndrome (IBS)	45.0	NDDIC
Anxiety Disorders	40.0	NIMH
Migraine Headaches	36.0	MRF
Restless Leg Syndrome (RLS)	31.5	NIH
Raynaud's Syndrome	28.0	RO
Depression	23.8	NIMH
Gluten Sensitivities/Neuropathies	20.0	msa
Multiple Chemical Sensitivities (MCS)	19.0	msa
Attention Deficit Disorder (ADHD)	17.0	msa
Interstitial Cystitis/Bladder Pain	10.0	JUCC
Eating Disorders	8.0	SCDMH
Fibromyalgia	6.0	ACR
Electromagnetic Hypersensitivity (EHS)	6.0	WHO
Alzheimer's Disease	5.2	AO
Endometriosis	5.0	NIH
Celiac Disease	3.2	UCSD
Complex Regional Pain Syndr. (CRPS)	3.0	VDH
Obsessive Compulsive Disorder (OCD)	3.0	NIMH
Autism	2.0	CDC
Irritable Bowel Disease (IBD)	2.0	NDDIC
Chronic Pelvic Pain Syndrome (CPPS)	2.0	JHM
Lupus	1.5	msa
Graves' Disease	1.3	HSM
Rheumatoid Arthritis (RA)	1.3	NIH
Cluster Headaches	1.0	msa
Parkinson's Disease	1.0	PDF
Chronic Fatigue Syndrome (CFS) (ME)	1.0	CDC
Connective Tissue Disease	0.5	NIH
Multiple Sclerosis (MS)	0.5	NIH
Amyotrophic Lateral Sclerosis (ALS)	0.3	CDC
Sarcoidosis	0.1	msa

(*See Data Source Legend & Notes on following pages)

* DATA SOURCE DETAILS FOR CHART OF MYSTERY DISEASES IN THE UNITED STATES

AO – Alzheimers.org.

ACR – American College of Rheumatology.

CDC – Centers for Disease Control.

HSM – Harvard School of Medicine.

JHM – Johns Hopkins Medicine.

JUCC – Journal of Urology at the Cleveland Clinic.

MRF – Migraine Research Foundation.

msa – multiple sources averaged (by the author, from three or more varying, reputable sources).

NDDIC – National Digestive Disease Info Clearinghouse.

NIH – National Institute of Health.

NIMH – National Institute of Mental Health.

PDF – Parkinson's Disease Foundation.

RO – Raynauds.org.

SCDMH – South Carolina Dept. of Mental Health.

UCSD – University of California, San Diego, Celiac Ctr.

VDH – Virginia Dept. of Health.

WHO – World Health Organization.

NOTE: *Chart A is not intended as a complete list of all Mystery Diseases. It merely provides a visual comparison of a select group of the more common and well-known disorders.*

SUBSETS &NOTES FOR CHART OF
MYSTERY DISEASES IN THE UNITED STATES

■ Anxiety Disorders as listed in the chart includes (but is not limited to) the following well-known disorders:

Social Anxiety Disorder (SAD) – 15.0 million
Post-Traumatic Stress Disorder (PTSD) – 7.7 million
Generalized Anxiety Disorder (GAD) – 7.0 million
Panic Attack Disorder (PD) – 6.0 million
Agoraphobia – 1.8 million

■ Depression as listed in the chart encompasses the following disorders:

Major Depressive Disorder – 14.8 million
Bi-Polar Disorder – 5.7 million
Dysthymic (Chronic) Disorder – 3.3 million

■ Obsessive Compulsive Disorder (OCD) was first categorized as a disorder in 1981 by the American Psychiatric Association Diagnostic and Statistical Manual of Mental Disorders (DSM). Originally thought to be quite rare, it now affects an estimated 3 million people.

■ Approximately 2.4 million Americans have Celiac Disease, and cases appear to be doubling every 15 years, according to numerous studies.

■ Once considered mainly a problem for teenagers and young adults, life-threatening eating disorders are now increasing at a disturbing rate in older Americans. According to a 2012 study in the *International Journal of Eating Disorders*, eating disorders now affect 13% of American women age 50 or older.

SUBSETS &NOTES FOR CHART OF
<u>MYSTERY DISEASES IN THE UNITED STATES</u>

■ The National Institute of Health lists more than 80 autoimmune diseases. Other organizations put the number at more than 100.

■ According to multiple sources, many autoimmune diseases – including Lupus and Multiple Sclerosis – have tripled over the past forty years.

■ A 1997 Johns Hopkins study reported that more than 8.5 million Americans were suffering from autoimmune diseases. Within a few years, a report by the University of Chicago put the number at 11 million.

■ The American Autoimmune Disease Association now states that more than 50 million Americans are suffering from autoimmune diseases in 2013.

■ Autism as listed in the chart encompasses all Autism Spectrum Disorders including Asperger's. Autism diagnoses increased 78% from 2000-2008 according to the Centers for Disease Control (CDC).

■ Autoimmune Diseases and Disorders occur because of an unknown malfunction of the body's immune system. As a result, the body begins to attack and destroy its own cells. Although there are conflicting opinions, many (but not all) of the diseases and disorders on this chart are widely considered to be autoimmune in nature.

One Little Pill

It all began at 1:30 in the morning on February 17, 1995. I was working at home on my computer, writing software code for a coal analysis laboratory. This was a programming gig that I picked up as a third job, just to make some extra money and to push myself a little harder. Perfectionists and workaholics are like that.

My other two jobs were full-time management positions, one in a university research department and the other as director of mapping services for a local data analysis company. Fortunately, my two offices were right down the street from each other, and my employers were great people, very flexible, and easy to work with. As you may surmise, I was an extremely busy man, typically working 80 – 90 hours per week. But I was relatively successful, fairly stable, and as content as an energetic overachiever can possibly be.

I was married with three beautiful children, and we lived happily in a large, two-story, brick home with a full basement living area. It was three floors of comfort located in the same peaceful, small town where I'd been born, and where most of my family still lived. I even made time, as often as possible, to shoot baskets or play football in the back yard with the kids and their friends. I'd never had any health problems to speak of, and had always been convinced that there was nothing I could not do, no goal I could not accomplish. My only apparent flaws were that I sometimes drank a little too much, and worked far too much.

On this particular fateful night in 1995, everyone else was sleeping soundly while I tapped away on my computer keyboard. With no prior warning, not even the slightest, subtle indicator, I became aware of a pressure inside my head. There was no better way to describe it at that time, and to this day, I still don't have a more helpful description. It was not a typical headache; it wasn't really a headache at all, at least, not as I'd ever known them. It was simply a vague uneasiness or discomfort that would not, could not be ignored.

I fought against the pressure, hoping it would pass, and soldiered on for five, ten, twenty minutes. But the mysterious distress worsened, until finally, I couldn't bear it anymore. Whatever it was, it was clouding my thinking, tightening my throat, and moving into my chest. Suddenly, I was scared.

I jumped up and paced rapidly around the house, my synapses crackling in my brain and my thoughts bouncing wildly around like a thousand ping pong balls tumbling in a clothes dryer. *What's wrong with me?* I wondered. *Should I wake my wife? Should I call 911? Is this all just my imagination and I'm totally over-reacting? Or am I about to die? Could this be a brain tumor or a heart attack? Or am I going crazy and completely losing my mind?!*

The main floor of our home had a circular sort of layout, connecting hallways that allowed you to make a complete circle if you wanted, and end up back where you started. I made that round trip more than 2500 times in those early hours that day in 1995. I knew this because I kept count of the number of steps I took, as well as the number of revolutions I completed. And to further help occupy my reeling mind, I alternated between walking quickly and slowly, forwards and backwards. I concentrated on making each circle in the exact same number of steps. And I did all of this until the sun rose and my wife came downstairs for breakfast.

"What are you doing?" she asked. "Didn't you come to bed at all last night?"

"No, I didn't," I answered nervously, continuing to pace. "I've been up all night."

"Why are you walking like that?"

"I don't know."

"What do you mean 'you don't know'?"

"I just don't know. Something's wrong and I can't really explain it."

My wife looked at me like I was crazy, and I couldn't really blame her. "You're scaring me," she said. "I don't understand. Are you sick?"

"No, no, I'm fine," I said. "I'm going to take a shower and go to work."

And that's exactly what I did.

I worked all day as usual, running between my two jobs. It was a fine day and I was moving onward and upward. I couldn't explain what had happened in those early morning hours, so I pushed it to the back of my mind, and prepared to write it off as one of life's little mysteries. I was certain that I would quickly return to my regular routine and all would be well.

I was wrong.

That night, it happened again – the weird thoughts, the indescribable pressure inside me, the odd dread of the nighttime hours, the fear that I was losing control. I was forced to get up and pace for hours until I was so exhausted that I fell asleep on the living room couch. In the morning, I was definitely concerned about these troubling developments, but took solace in the fact that I now apparently had a remedy for this weird phase I was going through – all I had to do was pace until I was worn out and could fall straight into dreamland.

That plan lasted about a week.

My thoughts became more bizarre and uncontrollable each night, such that pacing alone was not occupying my mind fully enough to maintain my sense of self-control. Sometimes I saw white spots floating around the room; other times there were dark shadows moving like demons and closing in around me. And I often had the frightening sensation that I was dimension shifting.

I began writing very detailed notes – a practice that I continued for several years – intended for whoever would find my unconscious or dead body, so they'd know what were the last things I'd done, foods I'd consumed, meds I'd taken, or any other pertinent information. Writing in this manner helped keep my mind occupied for a while, but it still wasn't enough.

One night I spotted a tennis ball the kids had left on the floor; and I picked it up and began tossing and catching it while pacing around the house. The two activities together made a powerful and effective combination; and, suddenly, I had a new strategy on my side to help hold the terror at bay.

I kept count of how many times in a row I could catch the ball without dropping it. I also kept count of the total number of catches, while mentally tracking my trips around the inside of the house. I'd toss and catch the ball left-handed one hundred times; then switch and do one hundred repetitions with my right hand. I did this back and forth, over and over again for hours at a time. Distractions like these helped minimize my distress by keeping my mind occupied, and provided a sort of 'comfort via computation' or 'calculation relaxation zone,' as I began to refer to it.

But it only worked for a while. After two weeks of this bizarre cycle, I was frazzled, exhausted, frightened, and very embarrassed by what was happening to me. My wife was concerned about me, and suggested I get some kind of help. I finally gave in and went to see our family physician, Dr. Kelly Pitsenbarger. That visit turned out to be a life-changing appointment that started me down a very long and entirely new path of self-discovery.

"You have what we call an anxiety disorder," the good doctor said calmly, after listening to my story.

I peered at him and said, "I have a *what*?"

He explained that my symptoms sounded like a classic case of hyper-anxiety brought on by too much stress or work.

"But I'm not stressed," I argued. "And I love to work. There has to be another explanation. I think maybe there's a tumor or something in my head, pressing on my brain and making me feel all these weird sensations. Don't you think I should have one of those brain-scans or something?"

"I'll make a deal with you," he said, writing out a prescription. "You take one of these the next time you feel the symptoms coming on. If it doesn't help, then we'll run some tests."

The scrip was for a little something called alprazolam in its generic form, or Xanax, as it is more commonly known. He explained that the drug was a member of the benzodiazepine family, and would provide a calming, relaxing effect by enhancing the activity of gamma-aminobutyric acid (GABA), a neurotransmitter which inhibits excessive activity in the brain.

His technical description and medical jargon meant very little to me at the time. I had never even heard of anxiety disorders before that day, and I honestly thought that his diagnosis was the most ridiculous thing in the world. I had the prescription filled just in case, but I didn't really believe that some little pill was going to help with what I'd been experiencing.

I was wrong again.

About 36 hours later, the symptoms came on strong once more. The pressure and pain in my head and chest terrified me. My vision was blurry and I couldn't think straight. My ribs were physically constricted, such that I couldn't get enough breath. I was certain that I was going to lose control of myself, or that something crazy terrible was going to happen. Random, absurd thoughts raced through my mind as I stared at the pencil in my hand: *What if I lose control and ram this pencil in my ear? What if I jabbed the point into my eye and shoved it through my head?* Terrified, I threw the pencil across the room to get it as far from myself as possible.

Trembling with fear, I took in great gulps of air and tried to control myself, tried to calm down. But it was no use; the thoughts kept coming. *What's wrong with me? What's happening? What if I get a knife from the kitchen and stab myself or someone else? What if I somehow hurt my family? Oh, my God, I'm losing my mind!*

Finally, at my wits' end, I swallowed one little, white, oval pill; and just like that, 0.25 mg of alprazolam went to work. Within fifteen minutes, a peaceful relaxation spread over me. My hyperactive nerves began to calm, my painfully-tensed muscles began to relax, and all I could think was: *God bless you, Dr. Pitsenbarger.* It was such wonderful, glorious relief from the terror that I literally wept with joy and gratitude.

Alprazolam saved my life. For a while.

Chapter 2

Danger Zone

From that day forward, I did my best to have alprazolam readily accessible at all times. I kept some stashed around the house, at the office, in my briefcase, and in my pants pocket. When I took a shower, I even placed a bottle of pills within arm's reach, right on the bathroom sink, just in case. And on those rare occasions when I somehow accidentally left the house without the drug on my person, I panicked big-time. To say that alprazolam became my crutch would be an understatement of gigantic proportions.

I did not, however, become addicted to the drug at that time – that would come later – as I was quite careful with it in those early years. My doctor and a few other people warned me clearly and repeatedly about its dangerous addictive power; and since I'd always had a healthy respect – some might say genuine fear – for all pharmaceutical products, I was never one to take them lightly. (Too bad I wasn't as vigilant about alcohol.) But I most certainly did take this drug as needed.

Unfortunately, while I was learning to live with my anxiety disorder and attempting to get it under control, my marriage fell apart. The full story of our breakup is a long and complicated one, and there is no need to go into the particulars of that here. Suffice to say, as with any divorce, both of us had good and bad qualities, and both of us made mistakes. I take full responsibility for my share of blame for the divorce.

Sadly, by the end of 1995, my life was spiraling out of control, and the next two years were a sad testimony of a man who had no center, no spiritual foundation. I used excessive alcohol and sex with reckless abandon in an attempt to mask my anger, loneliness, and physical symptoms. As a result, my actions became increasingly bizarre as I exhibited a variety of psychotic and manic-depressive behaviors.

I became obsessed with the hair on my head, and started randomly pulling out or chopping off bunches of it at a time. I also began the disgusting and disturbing habit of spitting on the floors and carpets on a daily basis. I repeatedly trashed the rental houses where I lived, punching holes in the walls and breaking furniture and windows in the process. (I had plenty of money then, so I simply bought new things to replace what I'd destroyed.) And for some unknown reason, I bought three handguns and usually had them on my person or close by at all times – a Smith & Wesson 9 mm, a Beretta .22 caliber, and an old Colt 9-shot pistol. I had fallen into a very deep, dark hole.

On several occasions, that 9 mm was nearly the instrument of my own death. I remember often thinking how easy it would be to die from one quick blast from the barrel of that gun. I would stare into the cracked, full-length mirror I had propped up against the wall, and smirk at myself, as the Devil danced around me in the semi-darkness and whispered in my ear: *Look at you; you're worthless. What have you accomplished with your pathetic life? Why not just end all this misery? Do it.*

His putrid, demon-breath was on my neck, and his icy fingers tapped my temples. I leaned back against the wall and slid slowly down it until I crumpled in a heap on the floor. In my mind's eye, I can still see that cruddy, orange shag carpet that had probably been in that old apartment since the late 1960's. I slid the barrel of the 9 mm in my mouth, finger on the trigger, and stared at myself in the mirror for a long while. The weapon felt cold and slick in my mouth, and I remember thinking that I looked like such an idiot. Then the phone rang and broke the spell; it was one of my children. I am forever grateful for that fortuitous phone call.

The amazing thing, as I now look back on that deranged period in my life, is that most of the time I still managed to function somewhat adequately during the day at my primary places of employment. I credit that partly to sheer will power, and partly to those little white pills in my pocket, on which I became increasingly and dangerously dependent. But no amount of dogged determination could change the fact that I was struggling to maintain control as a functioning alcoholic or a half-sane madman.

I should also note that, oddly enough, during this time I was diagnosed with shingles, a painful reactivation of the chicken pox virus that typically occurs in the elderly, not in a 39-year-old man. My doctor was as surprised as I was! I presented with only a small amount of the shingles rash on my torso, but the strange tingling and pricking sensations annoyed me on a daily basis, and have persisted off and on over the years since then.

Still, while I did my best to move forward in spite of my assorted mental and physical health challenges, my daily life had an ample supply of flaws and failures, and I can cite numerous examples. At one of the International Coalbed Methane Conferences I attended – and where I was also a keynote speaker – I spent a good deal of my

35

time drunk, sitting on a nearby Interstate overpass bridge, throwing rocks at road signs. There were several other incidents when I shot my pistols into the air while driving along major highways. At least once a week, I woke up in surprising locations, sitting in my vehicle with my handguns in my lap, with no idea where I'd been or how I'd ended up where I was.

One of my more pathetic, but entertaining, exploits occurred one summer night at about 1:00 am. I was thoroughly and happily drunk, dancing around the apartment with Smith & Wesson, when it occurred to me that I had failed to properly introduce myself to my next-door neighbor who'd just moved in that week. So, with a vodka bottle in one hand and my gun in the other, I slipped outside while my girlfriend wasn't looking.

Wearing only a pair of ragged jeans, and no shirt or shoes, I banged on my new neighbor's door with the butt of my gun. When he didn't answer, I spoke in a drunken, sing-song manner about how I'd come to welcome my fine new neighbor to the block. I think I may have also serenaded him with the Mister Rogers theme song "Won't You Be My Neighbor?" I vaguely remember feeling insulted that he didn't have the common decency to answer the door when I was simply trying to be neighborly. After a few minutes, the door opened just a tiny crack, and he peeked out at me, obviously terrified. As I was trying to explain the reason for the visit, my girlfriend grabbed me and pulled me back toward the house, begging me to give her the gun and to come inside. I protested but did as she asked. Potential crisis averted.

But my manic-depressive behaviors and bipolar tendencies made this period in my life incredibly tumultuous, sometimes like a sad dream in slow motion, other times like some horrific rollercoaster nightmare. But the worst thing of all is that I still hadn't truly hit rock bottom. Deep down, a part of me foolishly believed that,

36

armed with alprazolam and alcohol, I would still be invincible in the end, and that there was nothing I could not do.

Chapter 3

Day of Reckoning

Thursday, October 23, 1997. 10:30 am.

It was a quiet morning on a typical day in the office building. I was at my desk creating a coal production database for a mapping project for one of our railroad clients. Nothing was amiss and I had no reason to think that this day would be different from any other. I'd had a big night of drinking and partying with my girlfriend the night before, but I felt no ill effects from that. Life was good! What could possibly go wrong?

And just like that, it all went wrong.

With no warning, I suddenly felt as though someone was reaching through the back of my head, ripping through flesh and grey matter, and pulling my eyes from their sockets. It took every ounce of strength and concentration to resist that pull and keep my eyes focused forward. I had the distinct feeling that if I did not keep them under control, they would roll back in my head, and I would lose consciousness and slip into a coma. I know it makes no sense, but that's exactly what I thought and felt.

At the same time, a pressure at the base of my skull came on quickly and scared the living hell out of me. My peripheral vision turned dark and my eyes went cloudy. I realized I was hot, then cold, then both at the same time. My muscles had no strength and I fell into the floor and began to crawl about. I felt the terror of impending doom as if all my bodily systems were shutting down. All of this unfolded in the course of just a few minutes.

Gagging and about to vomit, I crawled down the hallway, past another office door, and into the restroom. I don't remember how long I was in there, or even if I threw up or not. I vaguely remember crawling back to my office.

My boss, the owner of the company, arrived and discovered me in the floor, trying to reach the phone to call 911. A couple of people from the nearby office had seen me crawl by and they too came to check on me about that same time. They helped me back into my chair and talked with me for a few minutes, all of them suggesting I simply had a very bad hangover, some sort of bug, or one of my anxiety attacks. After all, I looked fine on the outside.

I explained to them that this was not like anything I'd *ever* experienced before. "Something's wrong," I told them. "Something is very, very wrong." I'd had plenty of hangovers, 24-hour bugs, and panic attacks in my life, and this was most definitely none of those things.

Someone had called my ex-wife who lived right down the street, and she and her boyfriend arrived within minutes. As everyone discussed what to do, my neck began making strange squishing and popping sounds at the slightest movement. Everyone in the room could hear the noises, and to use the common vernacular, we were all "freaked out" by the weird and creepy sounds. That's when they decided it was better to be safe than sorry, and

39

so they took me quickly to the hospital themselves rather than call for and wait on an ambulance.

The Emergency Room doctors and nurses kept me for several hours – I really don't recall how long I was there – and they ran numerous tests. And while I insisted all along that something was very wrong in my head and neck, their tests could find nothing amiss with me. They questioned me, of course, regarding my health history and asked if I'd had any recent medical problems. I told them I'd been healthy apart from two seemingly minor issues a month prior – a yeast infection for which I was prescribed some pills and creams, and a small spot of shingles on the back right side of my torso.

The ER staff quickly dismissed these ailments, saying that they could not possibly have any relation to the symptoms I was currently experiencing. Their opinion was that I'd apparently had one of life's mysterious episodes, the sort of inexplicable thing that happens to people occasionally. As you can imagine, I was not thrilled with that diagnosis. They advised me to go home and rest for a day or two, and assured me that I would be fine after the episode ran its course.

So I took a day off and rested nervously, wondering if my life would ever be normal again. The symptoms subsided a bit, though they did not completely go away; they simply became more bearable and manageable. Two days later, I doggedly but cautiously went back to work, still weak and with a stiff neck; and for the next few weeks, I operated as best I could in that condition.

Then things got worse.

Chapter 4

Into The Abyss

With each passing day, I was pummeled by an onslaught of weird symptoms, some seemingly benign, others quite painful and disturbing. I began noticing odd clicking and popping noises in my head, and a high-pitched ringing in my ears that often sounded as though a swarm of cicada had taken up residence in my cranium. There were also sharp pains in my sternum and rib cage that resembled the hallmark symptoms of costochondritis, a painful inflammation of the cartilage of the chest wall which often mimics heart pain.

My hands often went icy cold, while my ears turned bright red and burned. About once a week, an area 2-3 inches in diameter on the right side of my torso tingled strangely and became irritated for a few days, but then returned to normal. This was the same area where I'd had the shingles rash.

Occasionally, my voice would suddenly weaken to the point where it was difficult to talk; and then, just as oddly, return to normal the next day. Sometimes my throat tightened and made it almost impossible for me to swallow. The muscles and tissues in my face grew progressively tighter and more painful. And of course, my neck muscles, particularly on the right side, continued to cause me great pain, and felt as though there were steel bands inside my neck.

Eventually, this muscle and tissue tightness spread throughout my body, physically crushing me; and I often ached and trembled with weakness. My head felt pressurized and my thinking process was clouded. Some days, the least bit of exertion, like simply walking up a flight of stairs or playing my guitar, was too taxing for me. My ribs were painfully tight and constricted much of the time and I struggled to get enough breath. My weight dropped steadily until I looked like a skeleton – 130 pounds on my 5'9" frame. I was only 39 years old and I was certain I was dying.

Then things turned stranger still. It became increasingly difficult for me to go to public places like the mall or grocery store, and I grew frustrated and infuriated. On one occasion I determined that I was going to force myself to walk around inside the mall, come hell or high water. I drove there and parked, then sat in the car for thirty minutes, trying to work up the courage to go in. Finally, I walked up to the entrance, but could not go inside. I don't know why; I just couldn't do it. There was no logic, no reason, no rationale. I went back to the car and begged God for answers. *What's wrong with me? What's happened to me?* But there was no reply from heaven.

During the Christmas holidays, there was a big family gathering at my grandmother's house for what was to be a nice dinner and an evening of laughter and joy. My grandmother asked me to stop at the grocery store and pick up some extra dinner rolls, and I told her I would, of course. But once I was inside the market, the pressure in my head increased, and I began to shake. I fought through it and made a bee line for the bread aisle; but before I could get there, I lost control of my eyes. They vibrated rapidly from side to side, everything got blurry, and I fell down on my knees in front of other shoppers and store employees. I vaguely remember them talking to me as they helped me to my feet, but I couldn't understand what they were saying. Humiliated, I stumbled hurriedly out to the car, sans dinner rolls, drove the remaining mile to my grandmother's home, and lay down on her bed.

My family, of course, was very concerned and confused, but I couldn't really talk at the time, couldn't begin to explain what had happened. How could I when I didn't *know* what had happened? I was hurting physically, mentally and emotionally; and I was too ashamed to even talk about it. A bright, confident, and competent man had become a shivering child, curled up on his grandmother's bed, afraid for his life.

I prayed a lot in those early days of the battle against my strange ailments. I sought Divine aid and wisdom, but mostly I asked the Lord to heal me and make all the pain go away. With all my heart, I turned to the Almighty God I'd learned about as a child. I read my Bible daily, confessed my sins, and tried to attend church every Sunday and Wednesday. I wanted to be energized by the teaching of God's Word, and I needed to feel the love and support that comes from joining together with fellow believers.

But half the time, I couldn't even enter the church building because of my "anxiety disorder." And when I was able to enter the service, I had to sit in the very back, close to the door, so that I could pace in the lobby or run outside when the pain and pressure overwhelmed me. I don't recall ever making it through an entire service; I always ended up back in my vehicle. Sometimes I sat out there and pounded on the steering wheel in rage. Other times I wept and asked for God's help. I couldn't understand why He was turning His back on me. He knew my heart was true and my motivation was pure – I simply wanted to go to the House of God – but it seemed as though He had abandoned me.

For a while, I moved back in with my ex-wife because I felt I was losing my mind and I was afraid to be at home alone. I stayed in our 14 year-old son's bedroom on the main floor of the house because I feared using the stairs. I can clearly recall, to this very day, the terror and hopelessness that possessed me during that time. I distinctly remember begging God to help me, to save me, to show me what to do. My tears literally soaked the pillow and my arms were so weak I could barely lift them. I was staring into the abyss.

But in that moment when I felt as though I could not go on, something miraculous happened. The faces of my three beautiful children appeared before me, and I slowly scribbled their names – *Ashley, Michael, Meagan* – on a sheet of paper. I wrote nothing else, just those three names. For hours, I lay there with that page clutched to my chest, and allowed my mind to wander the landscapes of my children's lives.

I saw our precious first-born, Ashley, at five years old, standing at the end of our cul de sac, waiting to catch the bus for her very first day of school. Her golden hair gleamed in the sun, and her nervous smile melted my heart. Her mother and I snapped pictures, kissed her goodbye, and then wept like babies as the bus pulled away. We didn't know it then, but we were destined to repeat that scene one day, when that same little girl would board a plane for the Air Force boot camp in San Antonio, Texas. We were so proud. And yet so afraid. Only a parent can fully understand.

I saw our incredible, brown-eyed twins – Meagan and Michael – on the day of their birth. Six weeks premature, they were barely 4 pounds each when they burst into this world. Meagan came out first and immediately unleashed that dazzling smile of wonder. My wife, God bless her, was determined to deliver the twins by natural childbirth, just as she had with Ashley. But then there was some sort of trouble with Michael's positioning, and the nurses ushered me quickly out of the delivery room. Scared to death, I knelt down in an adjoining room and prayed while my wife brought Michael into the world. It was sketchy for a while, but Michael was a tough battler, just like his mom; and after a week in intensive care, we were able to bring both our babies home.

So much love, so many memories – all this and so much more flooded my mind, soothed my battered soul, and gave me hope.

I have to live, I told myself. *I have to live for them.*

God had thrown me a lifeline and I held on with all my heart, with all my strength.

Chapter 5

Doctors, Hospitals & Drugs - Oh My!

Over the next few months, I urged my ever-helpful family practitioner – the one who'd prescribed alprazolam in 1995 – to set up appointments for me with an assortment of specialists. I remained convinced that something had gone horribly wrong in my physical body, something as yet undetected; and I was determined to discover what it was and fix it, just like I'd always fixed everything else in my life.

First, he scheduled me for a thorough, two-day exam at the highly respected Greenbrier Medical Clinic in Lewisburg, WV. There they checked me over, ran all sorts of tests, and found nothing wrong. They suggested I seek counseling. This was not, by the way, the first time I'd heard this suggestion, nor would it be the last.

Second, my good doctor pulled some strings and got me in to see world-renowned Dr. John Jane, the neurosurgeon who attended to the famous actor, Christopher "Superman" Reeve, after his devastating spinal break. Dr. Jane and his team at the University of

Virginia Hospital examined, scanned and tested me for two days, but the result was the same. Dr. Jane was kind yet firm as he informed me that my films appeared to be fairly clean and he could see nothing to indicate a physical problem. And he too suggested I consider making an appointment with a psychologist or psychiatrist.

All in all, from 1997-1999, I was examined by a bevy of doctors, neurologists, neurosurgeons, cardiologists, pulmonologists, endocrinologists, and a host of others. I traveled all over the eastern United States for EKGs, EMGs, MRIs, cat-scans, x-rays, ultrasounds, blood work, stress tests, and various other examinations I can't even begin to recall.

All results came back within the normal range, other than a slight mitral valve prolapse problem with my heart, and some minor degeneration in vertebrae C4 and C5. I was told repeatedly that these problems were not uncommon for a man my age, and could not cause the symptoms I was describing. I can't tell you how many doctors rolled their eyes at me and smugly dismissed my story and list of symptoms.

During this time, I also made many unexpected visits to the hospital in addition to my scheduled appointments. My overwhelming panic sometimes forced me to the Emergency Room. As much as I disliked being inside any medical facility, I began to look at the ER as a sort of refuge, a place where they would attempt to care for me should the unthinkable – whatever that might be – happen. By this time, my oldest daughter had her driver's license; and I'm ashamed to admit it now, but I had her take me to the Emergency Room on a few occasions when I was certain I was having a heart attack, suffering a stroke, or going insane. As soon as we'd get in the car, I'd feel a little better, just knowing we were on the way to a safer place. Then, I'd feel a surge of relief when we arrived at the hospital and went inside.

Some of my unexpected doctor visits were due to the feeling that I was going blind! My vision became fuzzy and blurred at times, and it seemed as though I was peering through a hazy tunnel. Fluorescein angiograms revealed that I was experiencing significant central retinal vein occlusions in my left eye, but no cause could ever be determined.

Throughout the course of my many varied struggles, several doctors suggested I try an antidepressant medication. Some physicians prodded me gently in this direction, while others urged me strongly, even resorting to scare tactics. But all of them extolled the many virtues of these various mood-altering, neurotransmitter-manipulating, mystery medications. I use the word "mystery" because no one really knows how or why these pharmaceutical products sometimes appear to help some people.

I must confess here that I was biased on this topic from the very beginning. I was raised to be a drinker in a family of drinkers. After all, my grandfather owned a beer distributing company. Alcohol I understood; pharmaceuticals I did not. So, if I was going to self-medicate, I preferred to use my familiar, tried-and-true drugs of choice: vodka and beer. These were my old friends; I knew them well and trusted them completely. Besides, I further reasoned, humans have been indulging in the pleasures of alcohol for nearly as long as there have been humans.

In my opinion, taking mood-altering chemicals cranked out by the big drug-makers is like playing Russian roulette with your brain chemicals. And often, those who take them become zombie-like shells of who they once were. The medical community admits, directly on the packaging of these products, that these drugs *seem* to affect serotonin, norepinephrine, and dopamine in the human body, *in ways that no one understands*. They further print on the labels a list of frightening side effects – including hallucinations, seizures and suicide – as long as a horse's leg!

It should be noted, of course, that these drugs can in some cases be life-savers and difference-makers for people with debilitating symptoms, who have tried a variety of other treatments with no improvement.

Several antidepressants were prescribed for me between 1998 and 2001, and I confess that I tried some of them, in spite of my admitted misgivings. I still retained a fair measure of faith in doctors at the time, and so I was sometimes persuaded by their very convincing arguments as to why an antidepressant would help me. But as they say on television commercials: *Your results may vary*. And mine most certainly did.

I do not pretend to speak as a medical professional, nor do I claim to have first-hand knowledge of all SSRI, SNRI, Tricyclic, and Tetracyclic antidepressants. But I can speak with authority regarding *my direct experience* with some of these drugs – either from taking them myself or by seeing their effects on loved ones and friends.

Within an hour of taking my first dose of Serzone, I was in agony. Excruciating pain shot through my body, and I felt as though I was being ripped apart. Luvox terrified me by turning me into a mindless zombie in the span of three days. Paxil caused disturbing physical spasms for four weeks until I stopped taking it. I tolerated Zoloft for a few months with no visible side effects, but it did absolutely nothing for me.

Amitriptyline, Lexapro, Prozac, Wellbutrin, and Effexor were also prescribed for me at one time or another, but I decided against taking them. There may be people who have been helped by these particular pharmaceuticals, but I'd seen the devastation they had caused in other people near and dear to me.

In my ongoing search for answers to my medical mysteries and the cause of my strange symptoms, I also looked at many of the more unusual possibilities. I had the house checked for mold, and also monitored for radon, carbon monoxide, and other dangerous gases. I investigated the possible effects and dangers of the toner used in our electrostatic printer-plotter at the office. Rheumatologists drew 15-20 vials of blood per visit to check for immuno-related markers that might indicate Lyme disease from a tick bite or other rare illnesses or disorders. My dentist checked me for Temporal Mandibular Joint Disorder (TMJ), and though he found little sign of a problem, he fitted me with a mouth guard just to be on the safe side. Finally, several audiologists put me through an extensive battery of ear and vestibular tests which confirmed marked hearing loss and tinnitus, but nothing else.

Apparently, the problem really was all in my head.

Chapter 6

All In My Head

I had tried everything that made sense to me, and come up with zero answers or solutions. I was at the end of my rope, angry and frustrated, but I wasn't about to give up. Though I certainly did not believe for one second that my problems were actually psychological or that I needed to see a counselor, I was still willing to give it a try. My thinking was: *Alright then, if they want me to talk to someone, then I'll talk to someone.* Dr. Pitsenbarger referred me to a well-known and highly respected psychologist in our area, and so began a new leg of my strange journey.

I didn't want to admit it at first – with my less-than-stellar attitude and all – but my therapist, Dr. Charlie, was a fascinating and amazing man. A bit eccentric, perhaps, but I liked him right from the beginning. There was something about his gentle demeanor and stately, yet down-to-earth presence that was very calming. I suppose that's what you want in a therapist.

Dr. Charlie asked all the standard questions about my family, childhood and relationships, and we covered a lot of ground in the first few sessions. I explained that, of all my painful and frightening symptoms, the worst one by far was the fear that I was losing control of myself, going completely insane. I described the grotesque demon faces that I sometimes saw in my mind; they were half-animal, half monster, and seemed to be staring into the depths of my soul, whispering to me. I told him about the terrifying thoughts I kept having that I might stab someone with a kitchen knife or ram a pencil into my eardrum. Over a series of sessions, Dr. Charlie helped me understand the fallacies of this sort of irrational 'What-if?' thinking, and greatly eased my distress. He addressed the issue simply and in a straightforward manner, and our conversation went something like this:

Dr. Charlie: *Ron, what kind of person are you at your very core? Are you basically kind and loving, or are you mean-spirited and hurtful?*

Me: *I know that I'm a good person with a loving heart.*

Dr. Charlie: *And do you really want to hurt yourself or anyone else?*

Me: *No, of course not. I would never want to harm anyone.*

Dr. Charlie: *Then simply trust what you know to be true about you. Give no credence to those random 'What-if?' thoughts. Pay them no mind; they're not the real you. Trust in the loving person that you know yourself to be.*

I also learned a great deal about Dr. Charlie. He had been meditating for years – a practice I knew nothing about – and had even used the technique as a form of self-hypnosis to undergo ankle surgery without anesthesia. I was skeptical of that claim until I watched the videotape of the operation.

During the time I was working with Dr. Charlie, I also became aware of a variety of other so-called "new age" concepts and practices which had been completely foreign to me: hypnosis, acupuncture, crystals, massage therapy, re-birthing, past life regression, tarot card readings, yoga, tai chi, detoxification, osteopathic remedies, herbal treatments, mind-body energy work, and many others.

At first, I rejected all of these unusual treatment methods that did not conform to my preconceived notion of what was or was not possible. I had been a pragmatic businessman for years, and was the type of person who thought he could solve any problem by himself through rational thinking and hard work. I was a true product of western culture, medicine and mindset. So it was difficult for me to open my mind to the metaphysical realm and believe that these things might be more than just nonsense.

My counseling sessions allowed me to talk through much of the trauma of my early years, and to uncover and deal with my personal issues, weaknesses, and fears. To sum up a lifetime of sorrow and hurt in a very small nutshell: My biological father abandoned me and my mother when I was less than a year old. When I was five, my mom remarried a hard man who resented, belittled, and verbally abused me every day of my life. As a little boy, I felt totally and completely alone in the world. From the time I was five until I was about 14 years old, I pulled the covers up over my head and cried myself to sleep on more nights than I care to remember.

The strange thing is that, after living with this emotional pain for so many years, I'd convinced myself that my experience wasn't really so far from the norm. I just assumed that all fathers were cruel, everyone had a terribly unhappy childhood, and it was just all part of being a kid. But therapy helped me recognize that what had happened to me was most definitely *not* the norm, and that, as a result, I had internalized a tremendous amount of sadness and anger, and had been clinically depressed for years. I learned that there are actually many people who grow up in good, stable homes with loving parents. I had a right to feel hurt, abandoned, and angry.

The entire process was a wonderful, ground-breaking time that forever changed my life. Those three years of psychotherapy were invaluable to me, and I will always be grateful to Dr. Charlie for what I learned and how I grew under his tutelage.

The sad truth, however, is that therapy did not alleviate my physical symptoms. For all the good accomplished by three years of psychoanalysis, my strange litany of aches, pains and problems remained with me. Dr. Charlie could provide no magic bullet or miraculous cure.

Chapter 7

A New Path

I had gone to more doctors, clinics and hospitals than any man should; and I'd been tested, prodded, and poked more than I cared to recall. I'd been laughed at and dismissed by physicians; and even some of my family, friends, and acquaintances assumed I was either lying about my symptoms or had completely lost my mind. But I knew with absolute certainty that something had gone wrong inside my body, that something was physically amiss.

I had also researched extensively on my own and questioned anyone who would listen. I'd chased down every rabbit trail I could find and barked up every proverbial tree. And finally, I'd talked out and worked through much of my childhood trauma and buried emotions. But even with all these efforts, I still had no explanation for my mysterious symptoms. That's when I decided it was time for a new approach.

I began focusing less on finding explanations for what had happened in the past, and more on developing strategies for living a better life in the present. I didn't entirely give up on finding the cause of my health problems; I simply moved those efforts to a back burner.

Though it was a bitter pill to swallow, I began to realize that I might never know the actual cause of my symptoms, might never have the answers I so desperately craved and needed. So I did my best to take a logical approach and shift my attention to concrete things that I *could* do.

First of all, I took Dr. Charlie's advice and visited an osteopathic doctor for an assessment. I'd never been to a clinic like this one. It was in an old house with at least a dozen people scattered around the "living room," relaxing on worn couches and recliners. Most of them were snuggled beneath quilts or afghans, with an IV drip of some sort attached to their arms. I learned later that the IVs were feeding supplemental solutions directly into the patients' bloodstreams. The IVs custom-made for each individual, but often contained some blend of vitamins, minerals, hormones, glutathione, chelating agents, amino acids, sodium bicarbonate, and perhaps a variety of other herbal ingredients.

The theory behind this practice is that it provides a custom-made, nutrient-replenishing cocktail for each patient according to his or her specific needs: headaches, muscle or tendon pain, injuries, acute or chronic inflammatory illnesses, and a host of other problems. Delivering the "medicine" intravenously creates a rapid increase in nutrient levels in the body's cells, which, in turn, helps speed up metabolism and healing. Many people swear by this sort of therapy and healing process. But having a healthy respect for needles and any intravenous "cocktails," I was wary, to say the least.

After my initial examination, the osteopathic practitioner said that I had something called fibromyalgia. I'd never heard of it, but it sounded bad to me. He suggested we attack the problem aggressively – I was on board for that! – and recommended a strict, carefully laid-out diet, and three sessions per week with Kathy, his best physical therapist.

Kathy was an unassuming woman, small of stature, but full of energy and vibrancy. More than just a physical therapist, she treated her patients with a blend of PT, massage, and reiki healing techniques. As you might guess, I began the sessions with much skepticism, but Kathy quickly made a believer out of me.

Her technique was unlike any other therapist I've ever seen, and her hands were red-hot with the energy of her God-given, reiki healing power. She contorted and stretched my body in a wide variety of directions and manners; yet, somehow, performed her healing techniques so gently and so precisely that she rarely caused me any pain whatsoever. For the first few weeks of treatment, I was still rather embarrassed to admit to anyone that I was giving this "therapy" a try, but I couldn't argue with the results. Every time I left there, I felt better.

Along with the osteopathic doctor and his hands-on healer, I also tried several other alternative treatments including EMDR, biofeedback, acupuncture, and past life regression. EMDR stands for Eye Movement Desensitization and Reprocessing, and is an unusual but highly touted and widely accepted psychotherapy treatment method. In short, the therapist takes the patient back through his most painful memories and disturbing experiences, and then helps to ease the patient's emotional distress with a series of side-to-side eye movements. Some studies have shown that the movement of the eye as practiced in EMDR decreases the negative emotions and imagery experienced by the patient, by helping the brain quickly process and heal the disturbing memories.

This form of therapy intrigued me. I first studied it on my own, and then went to six sessions with a trained EMDR practitioner. While some patients have reported miraculous breakthroughs and immediate healing, I was not so fortunate. The treatment sessions for me were relaxing and calming, but there were no epiphanies or miracles.

As for acupuncture, I tried it with two different therapists in order to give it a fair shake. My sessions were two-part. First, small suction cups were placed tightly onto my body in various locations in an attempt to "pull" blood to the surface and improve circulation. Second, tiny needles were placed into my skin in an effort to relieve pain and pressure, and to improve my blood and energy flow. I found the cupping to be a bit silly, and my body just didn't respond well to being stuck with a bunch of needles. I'm aware that the Chinese have used acupuncture for thousands of years and that many people swear by its healing effects, but it simply wasn't for me.

Though I was skeptical, I also had a few sessions with a therapist who specialized in past life regression and repressed memories. This proved to be one of the most powerful and troubling experiences of my life. In the very first two-hour session, the therapist had me lay on the floor while she guided me back through my life, year by year. It was like slowly rewinding the movie of my time on Earth, watching it happen in reverse, but then stepping into it and reliving it.

When I reached the point where I was 4-5 years old, I became extremely agitated. The therapist asked me what I was feeling but I could not explain it. All I knew was that I was very much afraid.

As she gently guided me deeper into the emotions and memories of that time, I suddenly had what I can only describe as a sort of vision. I saw myself opening a storm cellar door, like those in the Midwest where tornadoes are common. I stepped inside, the door closed, and I was in utter blackness, a darkness so thick that I felt as though it was consuming me, burying me alive

There on the floor of my therapist's office, I began to shudder and shake uncontrollably. There were tears in my eyes, and I was moaning and speaking incoherently. I'd never experienced anything like it and I was terrified.

My therapist comforted me as best she could but I told her that I wanted to stop, that I couldn't take any more. She agreed that we'd covered more than enough in the first session, and quickly talked me back out of that dark place and back into the present. She said that I'd made tremendous progress by quickly breaking through to such a troubling issue, and that we could return to that point and begin there at the next session.

I was shaken and deeply troubled by the experience, to say the least, but my hopes were high. Having been so doubtful at the outset, I now believed we were on the path to a major breakthrough and resolution of all my health problems.

Once again, I was wrong. Though we had several more sessions, I was never able to get back to that dark place, never able to open that cellar door again. I tried repeatedly to make it happen, to return to that utter blackness so that I could work through it, and discover what horrible repressed memory might be lurking inside me and destroying my health. But I never got there.

Chapter 8

Snowball of Healing

Having been too long bound up by my obsessive-compulsive behaviors, anxiety disorders, and out-of-control "What-if?" thinking (catastrophizing), I decided that the best way to change my life was to replace my overly analytical tendencies and obsessive thinking with as many positive, healing activities and behaviors as possible. In other words, rather than sitting around thinking, I took action. I called it the 'Snowball of Healing Method.' Once you start a snowball rolling down a hill, it quickly picks up momentum, gets bigger and bigger, and becomes a powerful force.

My sessions with Dr. Charlie started my snowball, and I quickly added EMDR, osteopathic treatments, acupuncture, and repressed memory therapy. Next, with guidance from the osteopath, I made drastic changes to my diet by eliminating almost all junk food, processed foods, and items heavy-laden with "bad" fats, additives or preservatives. I lived happily and healthily mostly on fresh fruits and vegetables, rice, broiled fish, nuts, and some whole grains. I also followed a strict, daily regimen of supplements and specific "super-foods" as shown in Chart B on the following page.

Chart B: Daily Nutrition & Supplement Regimen

VITAMIN / FOOD TYPE	DOSAGE	TIME
Potassium	550 mg	a.m.
Magnesium	250 mg	a.m.
Vitamin A (Beta Carotene)	15 mg	a.m.
Vitamin B1 (Thiamine)	100 mg	p.m.
Vitamin B2 (Riboflavin)	100 mg	p.m.
Vitamin B3 (Niacin)	250 mg	p.m.
Vitamin B6 (Pyridoxine)	100 mg	p.m.
Vitamin B9 (Folic Acid)	400 mcg	p.m.
Vitamin B12	500 mcg	p.m.
Vitamin C Buffered Powder	500 mg	p.m.
Vitamin D3	1000 IU	a.m.
Vitamin E	1000 IU	p.m.
Biotin (Vitamin H or B7)	2500 mcg	p.m.
Calcium	500 mg	a.m.
Selenium	100 mcg	p.m.
Zinc	30 mg	a.m.
Chondroitin	1000 mg	a.m.
Glucosamine	1000 mg	a.m.
Fish Oil Omega 3	1000 mg	vary
CoQ10	200 mg	a.m.
Soy Lecithin Granules	7.5 g	p.m.
Flax Seed Oil	1000 mg	p.m.
Tuna, canned or fresh	4.5 oz	p.m.
Vinegar	1 tsp	vary
Cranberry Juice	8.0 oz	vary
Prunes	5-7 per/day	vary
Yogurt	6.0 oz	vary
Mixed Nuts	< ½ cup	p.m.
Apple, Banana	1 each p/d	vary

(*This regimen worked for me, but should be tailored to your individual needs, allergies, and/or other issues.)

Slowly but surely, I once again made exercise and physical activity a part of my daily life. I started with just a few minutes of stretching and walking for the first few weeks, and gradually increased the length and intensity of my workouts as I began to feel stronger. Eventually, I became an exercise fanatic! Five days a week, my regular routine consisted of one hour of very high impact aerobics, followed by an hour of weightlifting, then another hour of aerobics, and finally, a 90-minute, "cool down" session blending yoga, tai chi, and deep breathing. I did all of this alone, at home in the evenings after work. This combination of proper exercise and a healthy diet enabled me to stabilize my weight at 155. At my heaviest in 1990, I had been up to 200 pounds, and at my sickest in 1997, I was down to a skeletal 125.

When it comes to weight loss, most dieticians and nutritionists will agree that it should be an ongoing process that involves a life-style change, not a series of outrageous fad diets or new-fangled super-drink concoctions. It's important to find ways to stay motivated when you're trying to lose weight, but it is not absolutely necessary to join a gym, buy a closet-full of devices advertised on infomercials, inject yourself with dangerous appetite suppressants, or adopt a questionable food regimen you found online. You *can* do it on your own.

It's best to eat a healthy, balanced diet with a variety of leaner and nutrition-packed foods; while avoiding processed and fat-laden items. And as much as possible, you should include some form of physical activity or exercise to work in conjunction with your dietary plan. The two will work hand-in-hand to bring your weight in line with what best fits your frame.

Weight loss is really not a complicated matter; it never has been. Typically, you can lose at least 1-2 pounds per week by burning 500-1000 more calories per day. Eat less, eat smarter, and be more active – it's a plan that *cannot* fail. But like any other self-improvement behavior, it requires a great deal of determination and self-discipline. To improve at it, you must work at it, and commit to being in it for the long haul.

Along with correcting my poor eating habits during this time, I also reigned in my out-of-control sexual behavior by taking a one-year vow of celibacy, which I later extended to 18 months. This was one of the most empowering and liberating decisions of my entire life. Don't get me wrong; it wasn't always easy. Former girlfriends often stopped by the house, sometimes in the middle of the night, to tempt me and test my resolve. Some of them were passing through town on business, and I allowed them to stay the night on several occasions. We even slept in the same bed, but always with the understanding that there could be no physical contact. In almost every instance, those nights turned out to be wonderful opportunities for better communication and for building stronger friendships.

I did many things I'd never done before: rock climbing, caving, and mountain biking in local parks. I took a van full of teenagers – my three kids and some of their friends – on various weekend trips, including one to an amusement park, where I rode a frightening, old, wooden rollercoaster! I'd been terrified of carnivals, circuses and amusement parks since the age of 15. The crushing crowds of people, weird costumes, loud noises, flashing lights, and dangerous rides pushed all of my panic buttons at once. And don't get me started on the clowns!

I also flew an airplane. Dr. Charlie owned a small plane at a nearby airport, and he made arrangements for me to go up with him one afternoon. This was a big step for me because it allowed me to directly face several fears at once: flying, heights, being confined in a closed-in space, and not having control. I was nervous but excited, and I will never forget the joy and freedom I felt as we soared above the beautiful mountains and looked down on the tiny towns of West Virginia.

A cross-country road trip was another important step in my healing process, and also a very special bonding time for me and my children. The four of us, having never been west of the Mississippi, set out for California with no itinerary, no plan, and no worries. That one wonderful trip allowed me to discover my inner wanderlust that I had kept buried for so long, and it instilled the love of travel in my children's hearts.

During this period of my life, as I was rediscovering the wonder of my inner child, I also took up roller-blading. I'd never skated in my entire life, not even in my youth, and I was a bit nervous about embarrassing myself or possibly breaking a hip! But my children were thrilled at the idea of seeing their 42-year-old father become a "skater punk."

With Ashley, Meagan, and Michael at my side, I bought a pair of very expensive inline skates and strapped them on. Bubbling with excitement, I stood triumphantly for a fraction of a second before my legs shot out from under me. My hands instinctively reached down to try to brace myself, and I nearly shattered my wrists as my rear end hit the concrete hard. It was painful, embarrassing, and I felt like a complete idiot.

The kids gathered around, fearing the worst, and for just a moment, I confess that I considered giving up right then and there. But I didn't. Instead, I looked at the situation as a painful lesson learned. The salesman who sold me the skates warned me that I should wear the pads, especially the ones for the wrists. I should have listened rather than my foolish pride. So I put them on, got right back up on my feet, and learned how to skate!

In a few months, I was skating around town almost every day, and even doing some jumps and fancy maneuvers. Those skates were one of the best purchases of my life, and I used them until I wore them out and they literally began to fall apart. They're in my attic now; they have far too much sentimental value for me to ever throw them away. They played a big role in my healing journey, and all because I stepped outside of my comfort zone and took action.

Books also boosted my spiritual life and growth; and I ravenously read every medical textbook, spiritual guidebook, and inspirational writing I could get my hands on. I wanted to learn all there was to know about anxiety disorders and the power of the mind in the healing process. *The Power of Myth* by Joseph Campbell, *Man's Search for Meaning* by Viktor E. Frankl, and *Feel the Fear and Do It Anyway* by Susan Jeffers were three of my personal favorites that played a vital role in my life's journey.

Gradually, with all the changes I was making on a daily basis, I began to see things more clearly and to understand that my life was not about how much money I made, how many possessions I owned, or what worldly goals I was able to accomplish. I made a daily, conscious effort to slow down considerably, cut back on my workload, and change the way I interacted with other people and with the world itself.

I learned that if I filled my life with positive activities, there was less time for negative ones. It was basic math! I discovered that it's not easy to worry, fear, or be sad when my mind and body are fully engaged in flying a plane, learning to skate, meeting new people at a coffeehouse open mic night, reading an inspirational book, or standing on the edge of the Grand Canyon.

Instead of lunching with business colleagues and drinking shots of vodka, I took leisurely midday walks in the sunshine. Instead of talking *at* people about all my big plans for the future or my complaints with the world, I conversed *with* them about the good things in life. Other times, I simply kept quiet and listened to the Earth. I often walked in the woods and heard the whisper of the wind through the trees. I soaked in the sounds of chirping birds, chattering squirrels, croaking frogs, and leaves and twigs crunching underfoot. I began to see myself for what I truly was – just one small but special part of God's marvelous creation.

Chapter 9

Meditate On That!

As a man thinketh in his heart, so is he. (Proverbs 23:7 KJV)

A little stress in our lives is good and necessary. But it's been proven that too much stress harms us, destroys our health, and makes us more susceptible to diseases. Chronic exposure to stress overloads the brain with powerful hormones that are meant to be activated only for short-term situations. This appears to kill brain cells by destroying dendrites located on the ends of neurons. Sounds terrible, doesn't it? Don't you wish there was something we could do to counter the excessive stress in our lives? There is.

Inspired by Dr. Charlie's example, I began the challenging and enigmatic practice of meditation, and it quickly became the most powerful part of my new life. I didn't really know exactly what I was doing or where it might lead; I just knew that meditation was something I needed to do. So I dove into the beautiful stillness and silence and began to swim.

Meditation itself is a paradox – on the surface it appears simple, yet it's shrouded in mystery. In a way, it's like concentrating on thinking about nothing. Or like emptying your mind to fill it with the universe, or drifting through time and space while never leaving your seat. But whatever you call it or however you describe it, a disciplined, prayerful, meditative practice will change your life. I cannot say it strongly enough: *Meditation will change your life.*

However, I won't claim it's easy to understand or to put into practice. It's not. Meditation is one of the most difficult simple things you will ever do. And since your daily life is probably complicated and hectic, you may ask yourself: *How in the world could I ever find the time or the patience to just sit still and do nothing?*

Self-discipline is the key. Once you decide to begin a meditative practice, you must set aside a daily time and then hold yourself accountable. It's just like so many of the other good things in life – it takes hard work, persistence, and discipline. But one of the amazing things about meditation is that once you begin to experience the peace and joy it brings, you'll be hooked!

There is no right or wrong way to meditate; it can be done anywhere at any time in any position. But I found it helpful to use a designated chair, to sit cross-legged as my position of choice, and to burn candles to foster an atmosphere of tranquility. I sometimes lit as many as 30 all around the room, but I always had one particular candle placed on a stool directly in front of me, no more than three feet away.

I meditated every evening after my workout, and gradually increased the length of my sessions from ten minutes to four hours per day. Eventually I was going deeply into a trance-like state, and staying there sometimes for as long as ten straight hours. By focusing on my breathing technique while staring deeply into the flame of the candle, I learned to slow down all my bodily processes and lower my respiration rate to one cycle per minute.

I also integrated classical music – something I admittedly had not properly appreciated before – into portions of my meditative practice. I listened to a wide range of composers, but the works of Mozart and Tchaikovsky were particularly spiritual and inspirational to me, and often gave me tears of joy and sent my soul soaring.

Some people might think of this sort of reflective quiet place as being such an empty, awful thing, a place where we are forced to let down our guard and feel exposed, vulnerable. For some of us, our first inclination is to run and hide from the silence, and to fill up the empty spaces with as much noise, clutter and clamor as we can muster. After all, isn't that the way of our high-speed, technology-driven world? It's as if we are determined that there always be something more to do, so much more to say, and an endless string of new techie toys and online connections in which we must immerse ourselves. We cling to anything and everything but that dreaded silence.

I speak from experience on this topic because I spent the first 39 years of my life avoiding the silence. It wasn't until my health problems knocked me down and forced me to stop that I began to see what I'd been missing. I've learned since then that the deeper I go into a meditative state, the more beautiful and the more welcoming the silence becomes. I know it makes no sense; I only know it's true.

I also discovered that sometimes it's only when you become very *very* still and quiet that you finally hear the truth – the truth about what you really should do in a given situation, the truth of what your heart really wants.

So, sometimes it's good for us to simply shut up and listen, because no matter who or what you're listening to or for, you'll hear much better if you just stop talking. Speak less, listen more. Sit quietly and you'll hear the Earth spinning and the Universe whispering. Be still and feel the presence of your Creator. Take long, deep breaths and pay attention to every single part of your body. Realize what a marvelous, miraculous creation you are! Feel the pumping of your own heart and the rhythm of your blood flowing out to your extremities and back again, out and back, out and back.

Close your eyes, breathe deeply, and notice the soles of your feet. Do it not just for a moment; rather, spend five minutes really *feeling them* with your mind. Think about all the places your feet have taken you in your life, and the wonderful adventures you've had along the way. Then dwell on the backs of your knees for a while, and then the tip of your nose. Pay attention to the insides of your elbows, notice your tongue pressing against your palate, and experience every hair on your head.

Then consider your brain itself. It weighs only about 3.5 pounds, is 75% water, conducts 100,000 chemical reactions in a moment, contains roughly 100 billion neurons, and processes about 10 trillion operations per second! Scientists claim that the human brain, *your brain*, is the most complicated and mysterious thing in the entire universe. Meditate on that for a while!

> *I am One; I am All*
> *I am huge; I am small*
> *I am Life; I am death*
> *I am being with this breath*
> *I choose Now; I choose here*
> *I choose Love; I will not fear*
> *I am weak, yet I am strong*
> *Filled with Courage all day long*

Those eight lines became one of my favorite meditative mantras – a Sanskrit word meaning 'tool or instrument of thought' – when I first began to meditate, and I've spoken it quietly to myself tens of thousands of times since then. I created it in my darkest hour, and I speak it still to this day because it calms me, strengthens me, and reminds me of the most important truths.

No matter who you are, I promise that your life will be better if you meditate. You'll be healthier and happier, and stress will do less damage to your body if you take the time to breathe deeply, and allow the transforming power and beauty of meditation to resonate through both your conscious and unconscious mind.

Chapter 10

Curiouser

and

Curiouser

It began as a slight tingling between my eyes, on the bridge of my nose. It was so faint, so subtle that I almost didn't notice it at first. But over the course of an hour, it grew stronger and became a quiver. It felt as though my face was actually, visibly moving in that small area. But when I got up to look in the mirror, it stopped. In fact, anytime I left my restful pose of meditation, it stopped. Then when I resumed meditating, it began again.

Weird. Very weird.

For the first week, it was minor enough for me to ignore, and I assumed it was some oddity that would soon pass, like a simple muscle twitch or the hiccups. But it grew stronger every day, and after another week, the entire area encompassing my eyes and nose was quivering and twitching wildly every time I tried to meditate. I became angry that my place of refuge, my greatest tool in my spiritual life was apparently being taken from me by some disturbing, inexplicable face-twitching force.

I hadn't seen Dr. Charlie in more than a year, since he'd declared that I was doing well, and that we really had no other ground to cover. But I quickly made an appointment with him and explained what was happening to me. Unfortunately, he said he'd never heard of anything quite like what I was experiencing. His best guess was that my body was trying to express or release something, or maybe sending me some sort of message. He suggested I find a way to simply let it be, to move forward with my meditation, allow the twitching and quivering to happen, and listen to what my body might be saying to me.

"Don't resist it," he said. "Just go with the flow."

"Easier said than done," I told him. But I gave it a try.

Day after day, I followed my regular meditative routine as best I could, but the face-twitching intensified. For months I listened to my body and asked God to reveal to me what was happening, to show me what I needed to do. But once again, there were no answers.

The twitching spread and turned into a frightening upper body spasm. However, I did not resist it; instead, I let it happen and did my best to be fully present in the moment with it. Every day the spasms would take control of me as if an electrical sort of power was shooting up and down my spine. If I was lying down, it caused my upper body to repeatedly and spasmodically jerk up off the bed, and I often groaned or screamed out in anguish. My face would contort into hideous expressions of pain as all the muscles in my body locked up as though trapped in a steel vise. It seemed like something unspeakable was inside me, attempting to tear my flesh apart and rip its way out of the deepest recesses of my being. This sometimes went on for hours and it could be terrifying.

Of course, I told no one other than Dr. Charlie about any of this at the time because I was extremely embarrassed and felt like some kind of freak. After all, I'd never heard of anyone in my entire life who had experienced something that seemed to me to be so outrageously absurd. And, after having made such great progress with my health and spiritual life, I was angry that God or the Universe was apparently taking it all away from me for some unknown reason.

Chapter 11

Change Is Strange

To everything there is a season, and a time to every purpose under the heaven: a time to be born, and a time to die; a time to plant, and a time to pluck up that which is planted. (Ecclesiastes 3:1-2 KJV)

The next four years of my life were jam-packed with more changes and stress than anything I ever could have imagined. First, my ex-wife and I remarried – for the third time! Then, as if that major life change wasn't enough, we decided to resign from our jobs, cash in our savings accounts, and sell our houses. A few months later, when the children graduated from high school and joined the Air Force, she and I set off for Nashville, TN, so that I could pursue my secret passion and lifelong dream to be a songwriter.

Our money lasted for about two years, but unfortunately, the marriage did not. (That's a long story for another time, but after three failed attempts, no one can say that the two of us didn't make every effort to find marital bliss. We remain good friends to this day.) After the divorce, my ex-wife moved away from Nashville, and

I took part-time work where I could find it. I wrote songs, performed, and played the role of starving artist.

During this entire period, all of my strange symptoms – including the newest ones, the freakish face twitching and body spasms – remained with me on a daily basis. Even with all the changes I'd made to improve my diet, attitude, lifestyle, and overall health, my painful physical symptoms never left me, not even for one single day. But the many things I'd learned and put into practice did help to ease my pain and suffering, generally improve my health, and help me manage my anxiety disorders, panic attacks, obsessive compulsive disorder, depression, agoraphobia, and fibromyalgia.

So, as I settled into my new life in Nashville, I continued with my various dietary, spiritual and meditative practices. However, as you might imagine, I was no longer able to devote 12 hours per day to being some sort of guru. I had taken a big risk to leave my old life behind, and I was on my own, following my dream in Music City. It was a challenging but wonderful time, even with my health issues.

Then something surprising happened: I fell in love with someone I met on Match.com. She was a deeply spiritual woman, open-minded to all the possibilities of the Universe, and she became the first person, other than my therapists, with whom I truly shared all of the intimate and embarrassing details of my strange health problems, including the face twitching and body spasms.

We married in 2003 and began our glorious journey together. Many times, she laid her healing hands upon me and bore silent witness as I experienced the pain, twitching and spasms. She gave comfort and support at all times, and helped me to open up and face my illnesses without embarrassment.

That was a crucial matter for me: the shame and humiliation I felt about having such vague and seemingly benign health problems. From my perspective, I'd always felt that people were looking down on me, viewing me as weak. Anxiety disorders don't carry the same weight as all the "big-name" diseases. Panic attacks don't have the mojo of a stroke. Agoraphobia is an impressive-sounding word, but it's nothing compared to the C-word, cancer. Tell someone you had a heart attack, and that gets their attention and respect right away. But tell them you have anxiety problems, and they often give you the eye-rolling treatment. Inform them that you have chronic fatigue syndrome, and you might hear them say something like this: "Yeah, well, everybody gets tired, buddy. You just got to learn to tough it out."

When I think of having an anxiety disorder, in my mind I hear my stepfather's voice calling me *weak, sissy, pansy, little girl*, and numerous other things much too vulgar and filthy to mention here. As a result, for me, having these mysterious disorders was an embarrassment, an example of my weakness. That's why, in the beginning, I would marshal my forces, gather my inner strength and determine that I would overcome on my own through sheer determination. For a few days I would win some battles and feel good about myself; but eventually the little demons would come back. Even now, with all the progress I've made over the years, they always come back.

Chapter 12

Chocolate Cake!

March 6, 2006.

The only thing different about this typical Monday afternoon was that, just for the fun of it, I decided to try my hand at baking a chocolate cake with chocolate icing. I'd rarely made a cake in my life, and certainly not in years, not since the kids were young. I wasn't sure I could even do it successfully, but it turned out pretty well. I celebrated with a huge slice right after lunch.

Chocolate cake notwithstanding, I was troubled that afternoon, as I often was in those days, about the slow progress of my songwriting career and my ongoing, painful symptoms. At one point that fateful Monday, I became emotional, lost my temper, and had myself a good, old-fashioned pity party. I pounded my fist on the kitchen counter, and threw a spoon so hard that it tore a hole in a thick, metal cake pan in the sink, the very pan I'd used to bake my chocolate cake.

Ten minutes later, I had to go to the bathroom. When I sat down on the toilet, there was a huge liquid release from my bowels into the bowl. The sound of it alone was shocking, but nothing compared to the sight. The toilet was full of blood.

Don't panic, I told myself. *It's probably just a really bad hemorrhoid.* I'd had one of those once that bled a fair amount – although nothing like this – and I desperately wanted to believe that's what this was. I certainly didn't want to consider any of the frightening alternatives.

So, like a fool and since I felt no pain whatsoever, I decided to rest on the bed, go into a deep meditative trance, and hope that the blood flow would stop on its own. BIG mistake.

Thirty minutes later, I had to go to the bathroom again. I sat down, hoping for the best, but the worst was what I got – another huge release of blood. I sat there for a couple of minutes and another gush followed. Fear.

I jumped in the car – this was probably not the smartest move – and sped to my wife's nearby office. I was there in ten minutes and explained what was happening. She, of course, like any rational person, suggested we go straight to the hospital.

"But I'm feeling better now," I argued. "I think maybe it's passed. Let's just head back toward home and see what happens."

She reluctantly agreed because she hadn't actually seen just how much blood I'd lost. If she had, there is no way I would've won that argument.

My wife drove while I, wearing my calm and cool face, tried to relax in the passenger seat. Within 15 minutes we were in our driveway. I opened the car door and stood up out of the vehicle. That's when someone turned off the lights.

I collapsed back into a sitting position in the passenger seat, but in my mind, I was a million miles away, gliding somewhere through a field of golden grain.

The sun was bright in a big blue sky and I was brushing my fingertips gently along the tops of the stalks of wheat.

But then, faintly, so very faintly, I heard my wife calling my name, felt her hand on my forehead, and heard the distant sounds of sirens approaching.

"Wh—what happened?" I mumbled.

"You passed out," she said. Her eyes were damp and there was serious concern on her face. "I called 911. They're almost here."

That's when things got really interesting.

An ambulance, a fire truck, and six uniformed men arrived and took charge of the situation. They had received an Emergency Message stating that a man had passed out in his car in the driveway. That's all the information they had at the time.

I was still sitting in the passenger seat of our vehicle. No one, including myself, had any idea that my underwear, the back side of my pants, and the car seat were soaked in my blood which had been released when I lost consciousness.

The paramedics asked for my name and age, and wanted to know if I thought I could stand up. I said yes. But when I did, I became woozy and immediately threw up on the ground. It was a thick black mass – the chocolate cake that I'd eaten an hour or so earlier. Only semi-conscious, I plopped back into the car seat as a paramedic radioed his observations ahead to the hospital: *We have a 48 year-old Caucasian male vomiting stool. Suspected bowel obstruction. ETA five minutes.*

Still unaware of the bleeding from my backside, they quickly lifted me onto a gurney, slid it into the ambulance, and placed an oxygen mask over my face. A frantic paramedic on each side jabbed needles simultaneously into my arms, desperately trying to locate veins to start IV drips. It hurt badly because they kept digging and pushing deeper into my arms again and again.

Meanwhile, I once again heard the crackling of radio messages going back and forth between hospital and ambulance about a patient with a severe bowel obstruction who was throwing up stool.

That's when the light went on in my foggy head: *They're talking about me! They don't know that was the cake I'd eaten; they think I threw up stool.*

I tried shouting, "Chocolate cake! Chocolate cake!" but my voice was muffled beneath the oxygen mask and the roar of the ambulance as it sped down the road. I tried to pull the mask from my face, but the men restrained me because I had needles stuck in my arms. I pleaded at them with my eyes and repeated my chocolate cake refrain, but they just didn't understand. One of the paramedics patted my arm, smiled and said, "Sure thing, buddy. Just as soon as this is over, we'll get you a nice piece of chocolate cake. But you can't eat anything right now."

The next thing I remember was being wheeled into the Emergency Room where there was a flurry of activity, men and women in scrubs and white coats scurrying about and shouting. Several people lifted the pad I was on, and slid it directly over onto a hospital bed. My wife had followed the ambulance in our car, and now she was at my side, holding my hand.

A young doctor came over, prodded me with a stethoscope, and asked some questions that I can't recall. Then a nurse said, "Mr. Brunk, we're going to have to get you out of your clothes and into a hospital gown, okay? Do you feel strong enough to roll onto your side just a little bit?"

"Yeah, I think so," I said.

I lifted up and rolled to my side as best I could, and when I did, the nurse saw what no one else had seen up to that moment – *blood*, lots and lots of crimson blood. She screamed and jumped back three feet. Others rushed over to see what was wrong, and the place went into a panic.

"What's all this?" the doctor asked me. "Where did all this blood come from?"

"I tried to tell them it was chocolate cake," I replied. This answer made perfect sense in my convoluted mind as I connected the dots that no one else even knew about except me.

The doctor, thinking I was delirious, looked at me incredulously and said, "What?"

I tried to explain to him the absurd sequence of events that had led us to this point, but it was a long, complicated story and my mind was admittedly cloudy. Not to mention the fact that I was in a near-death situation, and there was chaos all around the crowded hospital emergency room.

My wife jumped in to help, and between the two of us, we explained to the medical personnel what had happened. They immediately ordered several tests and exams and determined that I was nearly five pints low on blood! The nice doctor said they were going to have to give me a transfusion right away. I said okay. Then he read off a long list of potential dangers, all of which sounded quite frightening to me. When he asked me if I could sign at the bottom of the page to give my consent, I hedged and hesitated.

"Uh...I don't know..." I muttered. "That sounds pretty risky."

I clearly recall the amused look on the doctor's face as he looked down at me and said, "Mr. Brunk, we have to give you this transfusion right now to save your life."

I clumsily grabbed the pen and asked him to show me again exactly where he wanted me to sign.

■ ■ ■

After five blurry days in the hospital and a battery of tests, probes, exams, scans and blood work, I went home with zero answers. No one knew why I had suddenly bled in life-threatening quantities, and no one except me really seemed all that worried about it. "This might happen again or it might never happen again," the gastroenterologist told me. "So go live your life."

"That's it?" I asked. "That's the sum total of all your testing and all your wisdom?"

"Yes, sorry, but that's all I can tell you," he answered.

And so I went home and did my best to follow his advice. But it most certainly was not easy. I was a man who had battled anxiety disorders, panic attacks, depression, agoraphobia, and fibromyalgia since 1995. Now I'd been burdened with the knowledge that I was a ticking time bomb, and that every single time I sat down on the toilet, it might be the moment of the next blood explosion, and possibly my death. We had no idea what had caused it to happen the first time, so how could we know what might or might not trigger it again? I was frozen with fear.

On top of that, there was the physical toll that the blood loss had taken on my major muscle groups. My legs were like noodles for months after that, and in fact, they have never been the same since that first bleeding incident. I'd never had any sort of trouble with my legs or feet before that fateful day; but afterwards, my legs trembled constantly and all of my shoes caused me pain except for one pair – the pair of Converse I'd been wearing when the bleed occurred. Fortunately, my wife scrubbed the blood out of them and salvaged them for me, or else I would have had no shoes to wear at all. Even now, on the day of the writing of this book, those Converse "Chucks" are the only pair of shoes I can wear that do not cause my feet and legs to ache. That too remains a mystery that no one can explain.

I was anemic for months after the blood loss, and my doctor instructed me to supplement my diet by taking prescriptions for Iron and Vitamin D, and by eating plenty of red meat in the form of steaks and hamburgers. The dietary change was a big one for me since I hadn't eaten much red meat since 1999 when I adopted my "healthier" lifestyle, as I've described in previous chapters. But under the doctor's guidance, my hematocrit and hemoglobin blood counts gradually rose and I gained strength over the course of the following year.

But recovering my state of mind, which wasn't exactly sparkling to begin with, was an entirely different matter. It was impossible for me not to worry about every bowel movement. In fact, anything at all going on down there in that general region made me nervous, whether it was purely benign or not. That meant I was constantly on a heightened state of awareness about my gut's growling or gurgling noises, gas, assorted pains and sensations, upset stomach, diarrhea, loose bowels, or simply the daily functioning of normal peristalsis. And, of course, all of that constant anxiety only further upset the delicate balance of my entire gastrointestinal tract. I was caught in a vicious circle from which I saw no escape.

Chapter 13

Nowhere Fast

I'd had my first real brush with death, and for a while, I had a very poor attitude about it. I'm not proud of that fact, but it's true. I had battled a host of mystery disorders for years, and now I had been given a life-threatening bleeding problem that no doctor could explain. Wounded in both body and spirit, I was thoroughly disgusted with all the dirty tricks I felt that God or the Universe or Fate had played on me. I was back on the self-pitying path of confusion, misery, blame and regret; and as a result, I fell into a deep depression.

I tried to deal with my problems by throwing myself into my part-time work and my artistic and musical endeavors. But I wasn't healthy or strong enough to work a full-time job or to totally devote myself to a career as a performing artist. Consequently, my life's dream of success in the music world seemed to be going nowhere fast. Sometimes I drank a lot of wine and wrote long, weeping passages of prose on my computer, and gut-wrenching songs of sorrow on my guitar. And although I did not revert to the out-of-control, gun-toting, vodka-drinking ways of my late 30's and early 40's, my outlook and my life took a hard edge and a bitter, pessimistic slant.

For the next three years, stress, worry and anxiety took a huge toll on me. Because stress is so very destructive, the more I stressed, the worse I felt in my body. And the worse I felt in my body, the more I stressed. This vicious circle simply served to make me angrier, and to further my depression, anxiety and pessimism.

All of my symptoms were in high gear. Every muscle in my body tightened and ached, my head pounded, my chest was constricted such that I could barely breathe, my legs quivered with weakness, my vision was blurry, my sleep was disturbed, my gut was in chaos, and sometimes I could barely form a coherent sentence.

In desperation, I jumped back on the doctor treadmill, and chased down every rabbit trail I could find, seeking medical explanations for my poor health, just as I had in the late 1990's. I visited at least a half dozen general practitioners, four rheumatologists, three neurologists, a cardiologist, a pulmonologist, and an assortment of physical therapists, chiropractors, massage therapists, and new age energy healers and clinics. In addition to large amounts of Acetaminophen, several doctors also prescribed various muscle relaxants and pain medications such as Flexeril, Promethazine, Tramadol, Lortab, Phenergan, Meperidine, Amitriptyline, and Hydrocodone. I tried them all and none seemed to be very helpful, and certainly not a long-term solution. There were too many distressing side effects, and the benefits did not even come close to outweighing the risks.

For a while, I visited a naturopathic doctor who specialized in Nambudripad's Allergy Elimination Techniques (NAET). This is an unusual, new age treatment methodology based on the theory that most of our poor health is due to allergies to thousands of substances – everything from eggs to aspirin to flowers to make-up to dirt – all around us every day. You name it, and they probably have it in a little vial, ready to test it on you. The practitioner supposedly desensitizes a patient's allergies by placing a vial of the potentially-offending substance in the patient's hand. Then after some subtle, hands-on energy work and applied kinesiology, the patient is theoretically supposed to become less sensitive to the substance and gradually stronger and healthier. This treatment did absolutely nothing for me.

Since I'd been diagnosed with fibromyalgia by more than a dozen doctors over the years, I finally joined a Fibro Support Group. Fibromyalgia is the second most common musculoskeletal disorder in the world, and its primary symptoms are widespread pain, incapacitating fatigue, associated abdominal discomforts such as Irritable Bowel Syndrome, chronic headaches, extreme sensitivity to cold and hot temperatures, poor sleep, incontinence, stiffness, and inability to concentrate.

I knew that there were untold numbers of Fibro sufferers in the world, but my local support group showed me just how terribly some of those people were suffering. One woman lay flat on the floor during the entire meeting because of the pain in her back. A second woman wept openly throughout the gathering, and another was so doped up on meds that she made no sense when she spoke. Attending those gatherings was far more discouraging and depressing than it was helpful.

My doctors, as they had numerous times, periodically suggested that I try one of the drugs – Lyrica or Cymbalta – designed for treating fibromyalgia. Eventually, when I entered into an especially dark period of extreme pain, I gave in and tried Lyrica. Because I was such a worrier, I refused to read the drug's warning label in advance, knowing that reading the list of side effects would cause me to worry needlessly and to possibly experience those side effects simply by the power of suggestion.

Unfortunately, after taking the medication for two weeks, I noticed troubling neck and throat pain – which, I found out later, was one of the warnings signs listed on the brochure which I had not read – and so I stopped taking it. After this experience with Lyrica, I once again decided not to try Cymbalta. It's very difficult for me to trust pharmaceutical companies and I simply do not enjoy putting unknown chemical concoctions into my body.

I tried a few chiropractors and each one had a slightly different approach. Some used the more common brute-force techniques of vigorously popping and snapping things around in my back and neck. Others used very subtle methods, even to the point of being so gentle that I barely knew they were touching me at all. Some of the chiropractors provided a small measure of relief from time to time, but for me, there wasn't enough consistency or noticeable benefit to continue seeing any of them.

I had a new round of standard allergy testing done which showed typical results – I was only mildly reactive to a few types of grass and spores, but nothing to cause concern. I also had several of my silver fillings replaced due to concerns about potential mercury poisoning, just to be on the safe side. And I went to sessions with two new psychologists to help address my various fears and state of mind as it related to my ever-increasing health problems.

My "germophobe" tendencies intensified during this period of my life, predicated by the helplessness I felt in general. It seemed as though my mind was "seeing" danger at every turn, deadly microbes hidden in every handshake, filthy germs on every doorknob, and transmittable pathogens in every breath of air. I avoided people, places and things as much as possible; and when avoidance couldn't be achieved, I countered the invisible army of germs with an assortment of weapons, including washing and sanitizing everything I could.

This sometimes debilitating condition is called mysophobia, an irrational, pathological fear of germs, dirt and contamination. And trust me, being preoccupied with an OCD-related fear of tiny microbes is not a pleasant way to live one's life.

For example, it is very difficult to hold your breath – for fear of breathing in the germ-laden air that others have exhaled – while shopping for groceries, buying socks in a department store, or standing in line at the Post Office. I often tried to inconspicuously pull the top of my shirt up over my mouth in order to filter the air as I inhaled it, all the while hoping that no one saw me and thought I was a freak. I wore a surgical mask outside the house on a few occasions, but most of the time I was too vain or felt too foolish to wear it out in public with no easily explainable or logical reason for doing so.

As these mysophobic tendencies continued to gain a foothold in my psyche, they proliferated rapidly and caused me to live in a constant state of fear, avoidance and hyper-vigilance. When signing a receipt at any place of business, I refused to use the pen offered by the attendant; instead I used the one I carried with me at all times for exactly that purpose. When opening doors, I used a napkin or tissue so as to protect myself from disease-coated doorknobs. In restaurants, I specified no lemon in my drinks because someone probably used their hand to place it in the glass. Nor would I use unsealed straws or napkins that had touched the tabletop, which, most likely, had not been properly sanitized. Eventually, shaking hands or touching anything that might transmit germs onto my person became an obstacle.

Chapter 14

EDNOS or OSFED

This period of my life also marked the rise of a related and equally disturbing health issue, a hybrid sort of eating disorder formerly known as EDNOS, which stands for Eating Disorders Not Otherwise Specified. [It should be noted here that reclassification of these disorders by the American Psychiatric Association will designate this disorder to be given a new description: Other Specified Feeding and Eating Disorders (OSFED) to replace EDNOS. This transition is underway as the new Diagnostic and Statistical Manual of Mental Disorders (DSM-5) replaces the old (DSM-4).]

Thirty percent of all eating disorders fall into the categories of anorexia nervosa or bulimia; the other 70 percent are EDNOS (or OSFED). Although not as widely known, this is a deadly condition with a mortality rate as high as 5.2 percent, higher than both anorexia and bulimia. Once considered mainly a problem for teenagers and young adults, life-threatening eating disorders are now increasing at a disturbing rate in older Americans. According to a 2012 study in the *International Journal of Eating Disorders*, eating disorders now affect 13% of American women age 50 or older.

At the root of my problem was a two-fold fear of food. First of all, I suspected that the food I was consuming might be the long-term cause of my poor health in general, or my 2006 bleeding episode in particular. Secondly, every time I ate, I worried that the food could have been undercooked, improperly handled, or somehow contaminated by poisons or pathogens of unknown origin.

Because of these irrational fears, I was hesitant to swallow when eating. As often as possible, I chewed my food excessively, held it in my mouth for minutes at a time, and then spit it out when no one was looking. This odd behavior was easy enough to do at home where I could simply stand at the kitchen sink alone and spit my bites out into the garbage disposal, but it was obviously much more difficult to achieve in social settings. In those situations, I would sometimes spit into napkins or excuse myself to the restroom. As a result of this practice, I wasn't taking in enough food to fully provide the proper nutrition required for my body to function as it should. But in my warped way of thinking, the risk was worth the reward because I was eating just enough to survive while protecting myself from a myriad of deadly germs.

I also reasoned that chewing and spitting out was a clever way to enjoy the taste of "bad" or excessive amounts of foods without suffering any of the negative consequences. With my method, I could have as much of my favorite things – chocolate, cookies, lasagna, pizza, ice cream or anything else, for that matter – without gaining weight or raising my cholesterol levels. I thought I was a genius! So much so that when a close friend suggested I had an eating disorder, I laughed in her face and told her she was just jealous because I had discovered a full-proof weight-loss method.

As I look back on this behavior, I realize I'd had an inclination and predisposition toward eating disorders for many years. A disturbance in my own body image awareness and a misperception of my body's size and shape always caused me to push diets and exercise to dangerous levels. As I mentioned in the opening chapter, this type of behavior is a common characteristic of workaholics and perfectionists. When I committed to something, I carried it to the highest possible degree. But still, nothing is ever quite good enough. Nothing is ever really finished or complete. Push a little harder, a little bit further. It's another of those vicious circles, and I've been trapped in far too many of them in my life.

Fear of one's own food is the ultimate catch-22. We must eat to live, but how do we eat if we're afraid the food we ingest might kill us? There can be no true peace of mind for someone suffering from this disorder.

I found that I was constantly bargaining with myself, thinking: *I'll eat just enough to survive, and pray that these bites I'm consuming are not the contaminated ones.* Under these conditions, anxiety runs rampant. And when you're anxious, your gut is usually the first place you feel it. That means you're ingesting food into a gastrointestinal system that is already in an uproar before the food even gets there. It's a recipe – no pun intended – for disaster.

To this very day, I remain in an ongoing battle with this food perception sickness. Rarely is there a meal during which I don't feel a subtle gagging in my throat or the turning of my stomach over something I'm eating. I may be perfectly fine one moment, but within seconds suddenly experience some sort of indefinable but powerful revulsion toward whatever food is in my mouth or on my plate.

Chapter 15

Return of the Blood

April 22, 2011.

It was 1:00 am and I was in bed, massaging my aching muscles and attempting to relax and meditate through the pain. Suddenly I felt the pressing need for a bowel movement. I hurried to the bathroom just in time to release a massive quantity of blood into the toilet bowl.

I immediately woke my wife. "It's happening again," I said, surprisingly calm.

"What? What's happening again?" she asked, rubbing the sleep from her eyes.

"The bleeding."

She jumped out of bed and we wasted no time gathering a few things together, including old towels and a bed pan for me to sit on while we drove to the hospital. Neither of us had forgotten the lessons learned when I nearly bled to death on my infamous 'chocolate cake day' in 2006.

There was little traffic on the road at the late hour, and we were at the hospital in ten minutes. She pulled right up to the Emergency Room door and I ran in to get things started while she parked the car nearby.

The waiting area was surprisingly quiet; there were only a handful of people in the large room. I hurried to the desk where one young man was seated behind the counter for patient registration.

"Excuse me," I said. "I have a bleeding problem and I need help right away."

He looked up from his paperwork and gave me the once-over. I knew exactly what he was thinking: *You don't look like there's anything wrong with you.*

"I'll be with you in a few minutes," he said.

"You don't understand," I argued. "I need help immediately. There's no time to waste."

His voice grew more firm. "I *said* I'll be with you in a minute. Just have a seat."

Irritated, I turned and looked around the room, trying to decide what to do next. When I turned back toward the desk, the young man had disappeared! I remembered thinking what a jerk he was, but before I could protest, everything began to grow dark. As I was losing consciousness, my rectal muscles relaxed and automatically released what seemed like a gallon of blood that had accumulated in my intestines. I looked down at my feet as I started to slump, and was shocked to see a dark red puddle of my lifeblood spreading all around me, creating a crimson circle about three feet in diameter on the white-tiled floor. I collapsed into it.

I faded in and out of consciousness as doctors and nurses got me up onto a gurney. I remember thinking how they seemed so friendly and efficient, hands-on and helpful. My frightened wife was at my side, holding my hand, walking with me as they wheeled me quickly down a long corridor. It seemed like we rolled on forever, and I remember noticing how the gurney made such a wonderful, rhythmic clacking noise as we moved along. I stared up at the ceiling lights as they whizzed by, and it was almost hypnotizing. The whole scene was so bizarre, just like something out of a television show or movie. But this was no episode of ER; this was actually happening *to me*.

After they cut me out of my bloody clothes, including one of my favorite shirts, the doctor explained that I'd lost a lot of blood and required a transfusion. I told him I understood and that I'd been through this before. Fortunately, unlike the paramedics in 2006, the nurses had little trouble locating veins for IV drips to replenish my fluids, administer meds, and give me blood. After I was stabilized, the usual battery of tests was initiated in an effort to locate the source of the bleeding: upper endoscopy, miniature video capsule endoscopy, colonoscopy, nuclear tagged red blood cell scan and maybe a few others that I don't recall.

But I do clearly remember the smatterings of bloody bowel movements that kept coming randomly for the first 24 hours of my stay there. I also recall vomiting repeatedly as waves of heat and nausea swept over me; and shivering uncontrollably when my body went ice cold, and the nurses piling six heated blankets on top of me to maintain my core temperature. And I remember the hospital bed being tilted backward – feet up and head down – at a thirty degree angle so that my remaining blood would stay in my upper body to better oxygenate my brain and other vital organs. And I also recall feeling terribly embarrassed as the nurses repeatedly had to clean up my bloody messes, change the bed sheets, and wipe the blood and stool from my rear end.

All told, I was in the hospital for four long, blurry days and came away with zero answers. As in 2006, the exams revealed only a few mild diverticulosis pockets – common for a man my age in western society – but nothing that indicated a cause for my massive bleeding.

The GI doctor said, "Sometimes an artery just bursts in there and we never find out how or why." This was exactly the same thing I'd been told in 2006 by a different GI doctor at a different facility.

Oddly enough, when I was discharged I had a completely different frame of mind from the one I had following the 2006 bleeding incident. Then, I had felt like a dead man walking; this time I felt like a man who'd been given new life. Somehow, within a few days, it was as though the blood they gave me had energized me like never before. I felt younger, stronger, and healthier than I had in a long time. I can't explain it, but I know what I felt. I even kiddingly asked the doctor at my follow-up visit a few days later if they had transfused me with Superman blood, because in some ways that's how it felt.

Still, when I went home, I was a mixed bag of emotions. Part of me was angry that God had forced me to suffer a second terrifying bleeding episode and another powerful reminder of my mortality and approaching death. But at the same time, the Superman blood played on my very edgy, angry emotions. Having been an erratic, bitter, unstable man for the past three years, I now felt as if I had endured this frightening experience and somehow cheated death. On top of that, I had apparently been the lucky recipient of some sort of wonder blood donated by what I assumed must have been a vibrant young man who drank a lot of Red Bull. A cocky, fatalistic sort of energy was flowing through my veins, and I was prepared to throw caution to the wind and grab hold of life with a pissed-off, reckless sort of attitude. I was energized, yes. But I definitely wasn't well.

Chapter 16

One More Time

Pain is a teacher that pushes you to your limits and pulls you closer to the Truth.

May 4, 2011.

Just twelve days later, it happened again. I woke up in the middle of the night, ran to the bathroom and bled massive quantities into the toilet. I couldn't believe what my eyes were seeing, and I was devastated. Completely *devastated.*

We hurried to the hospital, just as we had less than two weeks before. All the way there, I kept wondering why this was happening to me. After the bleed on April 22, I had decided that I could handle these random near-death experiences if they were only going to occur about once every five years. But *this...*this was less than two weeks apart! How could I live like this? Secretly, I decided that I couldn't.

This time, the workers at the hospital remembered us well, and they took me straight in for treatment. There was no grumpy person at the desk forcing me to wait, and no Keystone Kop-like antics by well-intentioned but misinformed paramedics. The same battery of exams was ordered but this time they included a new one, a scan for Meckel's diverticulum. This is a rare congenital condition found in about two percent of the population, which may sometimes cause sudden, painless bleeding from the rectum.

Because we'd gotten to the hospital and been admitted so quickly this time, my hopes were high for finding answers, but unfortunately, just as in the previous two occurrences, none of the tests provided any helpful clues whatsoever. Apparently, there weren't ever going to be answers to any of my questions. And for an overly analytical, detail-obsessed perfectionist like me, that was a very bitter pill to swallow.

The irony of it all was not lost on me. Just a few days before, I'd felt reenergized and capable of living out my last days with an angry, reckless flourish. Now, suddenly, I was once again a man in anguish. My entire body was in pain, I was completely fatigued, and truly as depressed as I'd ever been in my 53 years on Planet Earth.

So, on the final night of this particular hospital stay, I sent my sweet wife home. She'd been at my side day and night for everything I'd been through. She'd comforted me, brought thoughtful gifts to lift my spirits, and slept in a chair in the room with me. She was exhausted and I insisted she go home and get some rest. It would be the best thing for both of us. I knew she needed a break, and I needed some time alone with my Creator.

That night turned out to be the most frightening and important one of my entire life. All alone, staring up at the plain, white ceiling, I breathed in the antiseptic hospital air and didn't sleep a wink. Nurses came in occasionally as their rounds dictated, replaced my IV bag, and drew blood each time for further lab work. The monitor to which I was connected beeped softly beside my bed while the murmuring of the hospital droned on through the night.

I lay there in the dim light and spoke with God about my lifetime of successes and failures, loves and regrets. It was as if everything I'd ever done, especially my mistakes, all came piling down upon me that night. Even with all my best intentions over the years, and in spite of all my efforts to be a good man, I'd so often been guilty of being selfish, arrogant and immature. As I looked back over it all, it seemed as if I'd done more stupid things in my life than there were stars in the sky.

That night, for the first time ever, I fully understood that I was *human*. It came clear to me that I wasn't really better than most people, as I'd secretly thought for so long; nor did I have the inside scoop on all things spiritual or intellectual, as I so desperately wanted to believe. And no, I wasn't God's gift to women or to the world or to anyone, for that matter. I didn't have it all figured out; I didn't have *anything* figured out. I couldn't change one tiny thing about the past and I couldn't command the future. And no matter how clever or witty or charming or brilliant I thought I was, I could not make everything fit into neatly organized little boxes or compartments. The world was full of unknown variables over which I had absolutely zero control.

Suddenly the little demons were rushing into the room and peering into my frazzled brain. One perched atop the beeping monitor, one sat on the window sill, and one stretched out beside me on the bed and whispered in my ear. It was the same grotesque, dog-faced monster that I'd first seen all the way back in 1997. *Why not end this misery now?* it cooed, with strands of saliva dripping from its sharp, canine incisors.

Trying to ignore the demons and drive them away, I stared up at the ceiling and softly recited my mantras. But

I was deep in a pit of despair and, for a long while that night, I assumed I was not going to get any better. I imagined all the frightful scenarios where my health would deteriorate until I was nothing but an invalid, a burden to my wife and children, and would finally be put away in a nursing home to shuffle around in my socked feet and stare out windows for lost hours and days at a time. Since that would be the most unacceptable situation of all, I strongly considered ways that I might actually be able to kill myself without it appearing to be suicide, so that my wife would be assured to receive the insurance money.

I thought of a variety of suicide methods: shooting myself with my Beretta, overdosing on alprazolam, stepping out in front of a bus, or falling off of something tall. But regardless of the manner of my intentional death, there were two big hurdles that had to be cleared. First, it had to be made to appear accidental; and second, I had to be certain it would fully accomplish the objective. The last thing I wanted was to end up crippled or comatose; this was exactly the sort of scenario I was hoping to escape. Driving my vehicle off of or into something seemed to be the most viable option. If I did that, how could anyone ever prove it wasn't an accident?

As I pondered these morbid thoughts, the sky began to lighten ever so slightly outside, a dull gray spreading over the sleepy Nashville skyline. A nurse entered the room with an orderly, and announced it was time to take me down for my endoscopy. I was scared, exhausted, and beaten, with no clue as to where my life was headed as they wheeled me down to the lab.

They were preparing to administer the sedatives and start the procedure when I began to cry. Things broke loose inside me and tears ran down my cheeks and dropped steadily onto the crisp, white pillow. One of the attending nurses was a kindly, older woman with such a sweet demeanor. Like an angel, she put her hand gently on my shoulder, leaned in close to me and whispered six simple words: "God is on your side today."

It was as if she read my mind and knew what I was thinking and going through. Or maybe God gave her the perfect words and spoke through her. All I know is that it was exactly what I needed to hear. I closed my eyes and drifted away.

Chapter 17

Transformation

Do not be conformed to this world, but continuously be transformed by the renewing of your mind so that you may be able to determine what God's will is – what is proper, pleasing and perfect. (Romans 12:2 ISV)

Those last hours in the hospital changed me forever. Was I instantly transformed like a caterpillar bursting forth as a butterfly? No, not exactly, but the process did begin in earnest that night. I didn't fully understand it then, but my feet had been set on a new path, a better road. Healing was in my future, just not the kind I originally had in mind.

Physically, I was extremely weak for the next two months and had no choice but to slow down and take it easy. I was forced to do some serious thinking and to allow my trials and tribulations time to really work their way through me. Sadly, that's a very difficult thing to do in an age when we expect, demand even, fast actions and instant results. We want our food prepared quickly, we want to be served now, and we expect problems to be resolved to our satisfaction immediately. We are the people of the microwave, the culture of high-speed internet access, and the species that rules the world and blasts off into space.

But in affairs of the heart and soul, there simply is no substitute for time. Quick fixes are rarely the solution to anything. We cannot pop a pill and suddenly have great wisdom. We cannot stir some fancy powder in a drink and immediately have spiritual powers. Nor can we push a button and instantly be filled with patience and forgiveness. These things develop and grow with time and experience.

We may be very successful in this world and make a great deal of money. We might work around the clock to get all our affairs in order, compartmentalize things, and organize our lives such that we are the envy of our peers. And we could live in the finest house, drive the best automobile, and wear the most magnificent clothes. But even all these things combined are no substitute for being transformed daily in spirit and soul. Each of us must peel back our secret layers of pride and hurt, and reveal the true self that we keep so well hidden from the world. If we are not walking a spiritual path in pursuit of wisdom, love and peace, then we remain lost in the wilderness, completely missing the point of our existence.

Whether we want to admit it or not, there are questions we all seek to answer: *Who am I? Where am I going? What does my life mean? What is the secret of happiness? How can I know true peace, no matter how difficult my circumstances or challenging my problems? How can I love and forgive no matter how badly I've been wronged or hurt? How can I face my innermost demons, conquer them, and release them?*

Some of us hide from these questions, pretend we don't care, and avoid facing them for as long as possible. But these are the truly difficult issues that every human being has grappled with since the dawn of time, and we must face them, though there are certainly no easy answers. In fact, it's easier to excel in one's chosen profession, climb Mount Everest, cross a raging sea, or face the bullets of war than it is to answer these questions. And though the world changes every day, technology advances, and life becomes more complicated, the stages of human development remain forever constant. We are, in essence and at our very core, the same today as our ancestors were; and our outward battles are but minor skirmishes compared to our spiritual struggle to master our inner self and comprehend the mystery of our existence.

Chapter 18

Unseen Enemy

Pain is like a contrary traveling companion who tries your patience on a long trip, but makes the journey far more interesting.

How do you fight an enemy that will not show itself? How do you battle a shadow? How do you wage war against yourself? This is what it's like for those of us who live with the constant misery and embarrassment of fibromyalgia, obsessive compulsive disorder, depression, eating disorders, anxiety disorders, chronic fatigue syndrome, agoraphobia, panic attacks, and a vast array of intestinal bleedings and disorders. It's almost impossible to win an internal conflict when there is no clearly discernible foe and your body is an enigma.

Those around you can see the strains of battle on your face and see your shoulders slump from combat fatigue, but they can't see your foe. They don't know who your enemy is or what kind of war you're fighting. And there is no scan, test or x-ray that you can show them, no hard proof or evidence you can provide. All you have is your story of suffering.

And so, people doubt you. Somewhere deep down inside, they doubt you. And who can blame them? You doubt yourself sometimes. Your friends may not admit it or say it to your face, but they question your struggle. And you know what they're thinking: *He's crazy. He's making this stuff up. He's losing his mind. He's nothing but a hypochondriac. He's weak.* You know it's what they're thinking, because you think it sometimes too.

But we're not alone, and this is no made-up fairy tale. According to the National Institute of Health, 40 million Americans suffer from anxiety disorders, 23.8 million have a mood disorder such as depression, at least six million battle fibromyalgia, and as many as 45 million suffer from some form of IBS. There is an ever-expanding mountain of these and many other mystery diseases, disorders, and syndromes plaguing our society. But why is this happening? What is causing one hundred million United States citizens to suffer such a disturbing array of autoimmune, gastrointestinal, mental, bleeding, and musculoskeletal disorders?

Perhaps we should consider what we've done to our world and imagine the possibilities. Could it be the vast array of chemicals in our water, mercury in the fish, or the untold amounts of pollutants in the air we breathe? How about the hormones injected into our meat, or the genetically modified foods we consume? Or maybe it's caused by pesticides, radon, mold spores, or carbon monoxide. And what about all of the processed foods we eat, along with the additives like monosodium glutamate, artificial sweeteners, preservatives, food dyes, sodium nitrates, and sulfur dioxide?

Maybe the culprits are tainted vaccinations we've been given throughout our lives. Or our problem could be EMF, electromagnetic fields generated by countless power lines, transformers, power plants, televisions, computers, cell phones, microwave ovens, and many other man-made devices. Or, perhaps it's the effect of radiation from a thinning ozone layer, x-rays taken by our doctors and dentists, and the thousands of nuclear detonations that mankind has performed since 1945.

What if even one of the hundreds of conspiracy theories – poison chem-trails in the sky, for example – are correct, and our government really is intentionally infecting us with a variety of biological or chemical agents? And what about the incredible stress levels we live with on a daily basis, while being buried beneath a mountain of entirely too much information being received far too fast, every second of every day? Or maybe it's simply the deleterious, cumulative effect of all these things combined which is taking a deadly toll on our minds and bodies, and slowly but surely killing us.

Unfortunately, there may not be enough solid proof yet for any of these theories, or the hundreds of others just like them; unless, of course, you count the untold millions of people suffering from an ever-increasing number of mysterious symptoms and painful miseries that rob them of their livelihood, destroys their quality of life, and even sends them to an early grave. While some people may question the validity of our complaints and the veracity of our ailments, I maintain that there is most definitely something happening here, and it's something very, very bad.

Chapter 19

Revenge of the Little White Pill

In the early years of my battle against my mystery diseases, I was very careful about how much alprazolam I took and for how long. I would never allow myself to be on the drug for more than four months consecutively, and would judiciously wean myself off each time, and stay off it for at least three months. I'd heard all the horror stories – and witnessed some of them firsthand – about the dangers of prescription drug addiction in general, and Xanax, or alprazolam, in particular. Although, most of the time I continued to systematically get all the refills on each current prescription, just to be sure I'd always have an adequate supply on hand should things ever get desperate. Part of me still viewed that little white pill as my ace in the hole or secret savior.

But, unfortunately, as the years passed, my bleeding disorder and other ailments took a heavy emotional, physical, and psychological toll. I was often in a weakened condition, depressed, with a fatalistic outlook and reckless behavior. Eventually I reached a point where

I no longer cared much whether or not I was addicted to alprazolam. Having taken it off and on for years, I'd become less fearful of its power, and felt as if I could always keep my need for it under control.

And so I began to take it every day, several times a day. I took one to help me sleep, and I downed one to calm me when agitated. I also popped one any time I felt that familiar, panic-pressure in my head; or when anxiety caused my chest and abdominal muscles to constrict such that I could barely breathe. The little white pill was there for me whenever I had my weird, electric head-buzzes or terrifying out-of-body experiences. Soon I was taking more alprazolam than I ever had before; and one day it dawned on me that I'd been on the drug for two consecutive years without a break.

During that time, my health had gradually and steadily worsened and I had been diagnosed with ever more mysterious ailments, just as I had been whenever I wasn't taking alprazolam. In other words, it was clear that the drug certainly wasn't healing me; it was simply acting as a Band-Aid, masking my existing problems, and in the process, becoming a problem of its own. It was having a deleterious, long-term effect on my nervous system. I was shaky, erratic, un-centered and unbalanced; constantly on the verge of tears and emotional upheaval, teetering on a ledge overlooking a breakdown.

So, what good is Xanax really doing for me? I wondered. *I'm sick with it and I'm sick without it. Maybe I should just quit taking it altogether.* And so, I tried.

On three separate occasions I endeavored to wean myself off of the little white pill, but all attempts ended in failure. Each time, by the second or third day, I was a complete disaster, an emotional and physical wreck. And so, usually in the dead of night, I'd give in, pop a pill, and feel that sweet comfort spread over me. But I knew deep down inside that I was inevitably headed for disaster. I wanted off the drug but I didn't know how to do it. Or to be more accurate, I knew *how* to do it; I simply hadn't yet reached my tipping point, that moment when resolute will claims victory over a mountain...and then moves it.

And then I heard a story about a young woman who lost her life – one so full of promise – to the damnable clutches of prescription drug addiction. The message resonated with me, and suddenly, simply, sincerely, I wept and prayed. As so often happens in matters of the heart and soul, when the time was right, when I had ears to hear – to borrow from the words of Jesus – the truth was made manifest to me. I determined then and there that I would break my habit and stop taking the little white pill.

The first two days with no alprazolam were fairly easy, just as they had been the other times I'd tried to quit; but the second night brought with it a restless shuddering that disturbed my sleep greatly and caused me to begin to question my decision. It was on the third day, however, that things really began to get difficult. I became edgy, sweaty, and had trouble breathing; but I kept myself as busy as possible and soldiered on. That night I barely slept an hour.

The fourth day was chaos; I couldn't think straight or sit still. I paced, tossed my tennis ball, and counted my steps as my walls of determination started to crumble. *I knew this would happen*, I thought. *I can't do this*. Yes, you can. *No, I can't*. Yes, you can. *No, I can't*. Yes, you *will*.

On the fourth evening, the shadows leapt off the walls and screamed at me. Irrational thoughts of harming myself and fears of impending doom ran rampant on the treadmills of my mind. My restless leg symptoms were off the chart as electric bolts shot through my body, causing muscle spasms and tremors in my hips, thighs and calves. My brain wouldn't turn off no matter how hard I

110

tried, and the volume on my tinnitus was cranked up to 10, with clicks, pops, and roaring swarms of cicada. Going cold turkey off prescription medications is most definitely *not* for the faint of heart.

The fifth day and night simply brought more of the same. When darkness fell, fear climbed onto my back and bit into my skull. I ached from head to toe and shook with tremors as tears streamed down my face. The dog-faced beast returned, and stared at me quietly from across the room, waiting for me to surrender. *But I did not.* Somehow I found a strength I didn't know I had.

I yielded myself fully to the excruciating pain that was wracking my body. I accepted and embraced the fear that was pressing down upon me. I called upon my Creator God, recited my mantras and prayers like never before, and meditated upon the immutable truths of my existence:

I am a unique creation of the Almighty One. I am a child of God. I am loved and I am loving. No fear, no doubt, no worry, and no tension shall dominate me; for I am at peace with God, at peace with the Universe, and at peace with myself. I choose to say Yes to life, and embrace it exactly as it is, right here and right now. I will embrace this moment, even unto death, if that be the will of God. In love, I fear nothing.

And when the sun came up the next morning, I was no longer a slave to the little white pill.

Chapter 20

Perspective

Using the year 50,000 B.C. as an arbitrary starting point, scientists estimate that the total number of human beings that have ever lived on Planet Earth is approximately 100 billion. ONE HUNDRED BILLION!

So who died and made you boss?

One of the most important realizations of my life was when I finally understood that *it's not all about me.* Prior to that epiphany, I'd been foolish, short-sighted and arrogant; a product of our plush, pleasured and mostly self-centered western culture. Unfortunately, we have brought up several generations of humans in similar fashion, people suffering with a sort of narcissistic syndrome or ego-centric dysplasia. Is it any wonder we have an epidemic of self-absorbed people suffering with anxiety, panic disorders, and assorted other neuroses?

On many levels, our culture and the very environment in which we are raised trains us to believe that our individual needs, wants or problems are of the utmost importance and must be tended to immediately. We have

become so completely "me-centered" tha
sight of the basic truth that *everything is not*
I had to finally, fully understand that the wor.
revolve around me and I am not the center of the
Imagine my surprise!

In my opinion, many of our ancestors and cultures – Native Americans, for example – probably had a more realistic view of the world and their place in it. I strongly doubt that they were as arrogant as we are. I believe they had a greater cosmic awareness and spiritual connection with the earth, and accurately saw themselves in the grand picture as simply one small link in the Great Food Chain of Life. They lived off the land every day, stood side by side with nature, and understood the reality that they were only one wrong step away from being devoured by a predator or destroyed by a rival or enemy. They did not live in a luxurious land filled with modern conveniences, "second chances" and "safety-nets." And they did not teach their off-spring to count on a romanticized, last-second Cavalry charge to save the day in the nick of time, or that real life would usually be wrapped up in nice little packages, and neatly concluded for them at the end of 30-minute or 60-minute episodes.

But this is exactly how we have trained the majority of our children for generations with radio, television, film and all forms of media. We have done our best to insulate ourselves from reality. We desperately want to believe that the world is a great big, beautiful place where happy endings are common, everybody gets along, and we have a right to live in peace and total safety. All of those things are nice dreams to strive for, and there's nothing wrong with working toward them. But they are contrary to the harsh reality of life and death on Planet Earth.

The truth is that there are no guarantees for any us individually or for our species as a whole. An asteroid, a solar flare or some other cosmic catastrophe could incinerate the entire planet at any moment. An epidemic of some previously unknown strain of mutated bacteria could wipe out most, if not all, of humanity within days or weeks. Or we could destroy ourselves with some sort of doomsday weapon or another world war. All of these apocalyptic scenarios, as well as a thousand others, are possible, and some might even say likely.

Here is a way to put yourself and your problems in cosmic perspective. Think for a moment about the difficult – a very relative term – challenges you are facing in your life today. You might have troubles at work, a grumpy neighbor, a leaky roof, or a relative in trouble with the law. Perhaps you have panic attacks, the flu, Crohn's disease or cancer. You might have been injured in a car wreck or some other type of accident. Or perhaps you've lost someone you loved; they may have passed away or simply ran off with someone else and left you heartbroken. Or it could be that your problems are financial; you lost your job or you're overwhelmed with debt. Maybe you're homeless and hungry. The list of potential problems could go on and on and on.

But no matter the challenge you face, the harsh truth is that, in the objective eyes of the Universe, you are *not* special. Countless millions, billions even, of other human beings on this planet are suffering with a myriad of painful situations at every moment of every day. Of course, none of us want to hear this truth when we are hurting! We want God's full attention as we cry out to the heavens and beg Him or the Universe or someone to give us answers and to help us. We want to believe that we are at the top – or at least somewhere near the top – of the Creator's priority list. But just imagine how many people on the planet are suffering and crying out to God at any and every given moment. It's staggering to comprehend the numbers.

114

And we've only considered humans u
What about the thousands of other specie.
trillions of other living things on the planet?
live and breathe and hurt in their own particular
Don't they deserve consideration, love and mercy,
we do? Aren't they also part of the great family of 1.
creatures in our incredible world?

Consider this the next time you're wrapped up in your own situation, focused totally on your needs, and feeling sorry for yourself. Think hard about these truths when you are feeling overwhelmed by anxiety or the pain of your particular mystery disease. Just remember that, at that very same moment, right in the midst of your difficulties, there are also stars exploding, galaxies spinning, and black holes devouring worlds throughout the vastness of space. And here on our own little ball of dirt, while you weep for yourself, millions of other people are also weeping; or being born, hurting, laughing, loving, killing, starving, and dying. Not only that, there are also lions devouring defenseless gazelles, whales swallowing thousands of helpless fish in one gulp, and fires ravaging untold acres of plant and animal life, burning them to a crisp and leaving nothing but charred remains and ashes. Kind of puts a different spin on your individual situation, doesn't it?

We must face and accept the cold, hard fact that the world does not revolve around us, even though this is diametrically opposed to everything we've been taught by our narcissistic, hedonistic, consumer-driven, I-Me-Mine culture.

Imagine that the complete history of the world was written in a vast book, a monumental tome filled with at least one mention of every single creature – from humans to trees, dinosaurs to microorganisms, and ferns to frogs – that has ever lived on this planet, along with every single thing that's ever happened. Think of the massive size and scope of such an account, the grand picture presented by a record encompassing all of eternity. Then ask yourself honestly: *Would you be the central character in such a book?* Not likely. At best, you and I might have one line devoted to us. Our entire existence summed up in one sentence or phrase or word, even.

Depending on how you look at it, this may all sound quite depressing; but this chapter is not meant to cause you to feel as though you are meaningless and insignificant. It's simply meant to give you proper perspective, to remind you that you are but one blade of grass on the lawn of life, one grain of sand on the universal shore. Then, when you consider the big picture, your personal struggles and difficulties become smaller, more manageable, and your stress level is lowered.

Objectivity is the beginning of wisdom, and proper perspective is a powerful healer that changes everything. It allows you to release your anxieties and realize that you are not alone; you are but one out of a multitude of living creatures enduring similar trials and tribulations of life on Planet Earth. Pain, suffering and sorrow are simply part of the package deal of Life. This liberating truth will set you free if you allow it! Understanding this helps you get over yourself, makes your troubles easier to bear, and, most importantly, it's a vital step on the path to wisdom, peace and spiritual maturity.

Chapter 21

Me Love Food

We Americans love our food.

It should surprise no one that, according to numerous studies and reports, Americans consume food in greater quantities (an average of 4000 calories per day) and are more obese (34% of the population) than any other people on Earth. According to the Department of Agriculture, there are more than 200,000 fast food restaurants alone in the United States. And the Department of Health and Human Services reports that the average American consumes 152 pounds of refined, processed sugars per year, more than triple the amount considered safe. We daily ingest vast quantities of hormones, chemicals, preservatives and other food additives, with relatively little knowledge of the potential, long-term dangers to our digestive system.

Although we know the basics of the human gastrointestinal (GI) tract, our understanding of its complex workings is sketchy at best. We know that it is approximately 27 feet in length, and comprised of several major components from beginning to end: mouth, throat, esophagus, stomach, small intestine, large intestine (colon), rectum, and anus. And we know it provides for digestion of food and delivery of nutrients to the body by transference of food particles through the GI lining into the bloodstream. We also know that the remaining waste products are shunted along the pathway via the autonomic undulations and contractions of the intestines, until they are expelled from the body as waste.

But that's where our knowledge begins to falter. While we recognize that our vast array of human hormones work in unison to regulate every aspect of our body's chemistry – not the least of which is the digestive process – we are far from understanding the intricate interplay of the endocrine system and hormones within the GI tract.

A 2008 study conducted by the Stanford University School of Medicine made an astounding discovery: at least 5,600 separate species or strains of bacteria live in the human colon alone. While we are aware that untold numbers of colonies of bacteria take up residence throughout our digestive system, we do not comprehend the full range of their functions or their multifaceted interaction with the human gastrointestinal tract. What keeps this complex digestive system running properly? What knocks it out of its delicate balance? And, most importantly, why is it apparently being thrown out of kilter at such an alarming rate? People are falling victim in astounding numbers to IBS, IBD, Crohn's, Celiac disease, gluten sensitivities, lactose intolerance, malabsorption syndromes, intestinal dysbiosis (imbalance of bacteria in the gut), diverticulosis, diverticulitis, and a host of other autoimmune and immune-deficiency disorders.

Five years ago, I was not personally aware of a single person who was sensitive to gluten. Now I know scores of people, including myself, who are forced to go gluten-free in order to help control their gastrointestinal distress. Just take a look at your local grocery for more evidence.

Stores that five years ago did not carry even one product labeled "gluten-free" now have entire aisles filled with such items.

Likewise, a decade ago, I knew of no one who had Crohn's disease, lactose intolerance, Celiac disease, irritable bowel syndrome or any of the other GI-related mystery diseases. Now, not only do I suffer from many of these afflictions, but I also have many friends and relatives battling the same sicknesses.

When I consume gluten, I feel sick to my stomach and my gut swells up like I'm pregnant. When I consume lactose, I have intestinal pain, foul-smelling gas, and loose bowel movements. Spicy foods of any type give me heartburn, stomach distention, and excessive belching. And if I eat fresh vegetables or fruit, I have a pain in my gut and diarrhea within thirty minutes.

As a result, I can no longer have a regular sandwich on white bread, a bowl of bran flakes with milk, an apple, a banana, or even a simple salad! And of course, long gone are the days of pizza, chili, alcohol, cheeseburgers, carbonated beverages, fried foods, casseroles, or any heavy or rich foods. I could go on and on listing the things I cannot eat, but the list of foods I *can* consume is an extremely short one. How did this happen? And how did it happen so quickly? I didn't have this problem for the first forty-five years of my life. What changed?

Some suggest that humans were never meant to eat wheat or drink cow milk, that our stomachs weren't built for it, and that our bodies are finally crying out: *Enough!* Others say that we have poisoned and damaged our intestinal tract by consuming so many chemicals, preservatives and a myriad of other food additives that should never have been ingested by humans. Some say that we have disrupted and destroyed our digestive systems with "poisons" such as fluoride and chlorine that we've put in our drinking water. Many believe the true culprits are the fast food and junk food products that Americans consume in massive quantities. Others point the finger of blame at the overuse of antibiotics and at the low-fiber diet in western society. These are but a few of the many theories, and they all most likely play a role, but no one yet has a definitive answer.

I assert that our attitude toward food must change. We need to return to the concept that food is simply fuel for the body, not a way of life. Many people eat excessively when they are stressed, but food should not serve as a comforter for troubling emotions. For some, food is the most important thing in their lives, their greatest pleasure, perhaps their only solace. Too many people live to eat rather than eat to live. We must find healthier ways to deal with our stress.

Food is obviously a centerpiece of life; we must have it to live. But some people eat far too much and struggle for years to lose weight, jumping from one fad diet scheme to the next. Other folks are in a constant battle to consume enough food, to get sufficient nutrition to maintain good health. And many of us, those suffering from mystery diseases, face the daily challenge of finding good foods to eat that don't make us sick afterwards.

I suggest that you read food labels closely and become aware of what you're putting into your body. Remember the old adages – *Garbage in; garbage out* and *You are what you eat* – because they're as true today as they ever were. Food is fuel for your body, so fortify and energize yourself with the best possible fuels.

Keep a detailed diary of everything you eat, the reactions of your digestive system, any symptoms you experience, and the fluctuations and patterns of your bowel movements. You may be thinking that this sounds like a lot of work. It is. And it requires considerable discipline, but I assure you it can be extremely helpful in understanding your body's unique behavior and will greatly assist your healing process. (Of course, a food and digestive diary is also a highly effective tool for maintaining a healthy diet and for losing weight.)

By monitoring your food intake and by carefully tracking your digestive system, you should be able to eliminate many of the irritants, contaminants, and inflammation-causing items from your diet. And in so doing, you will greatly reduce your gastrointestinal distress and live a better life. I am living proof that it can be done and that it works.

Chapter 22

Gluten Gloom

In my late thirties, I began noticing a strange, red rash on the front of my torso, stretching from my stomach area up to my neck. It never went completely away, but some days it was brighter and more widespread across my upper abdomen, while other days it faded until it was barely noticeable. It itched a bit at times, but otherwise did not really bother me. But still, I would often notice it in the mirror and think, *I wonder what causes that.*

I also suffered regularly with bouts of nausea, extreme abdominal distention, gassiness, diarrhea, fatigue, and a general malaise that made me feel lousy much of the time. These various symptoms ebbed and flowed from day to day, but were usually present with me to some degree. Though they sometimes flared after eating, I was never able to pinpoint a particular reason why. Generally, it seemed as though I felt bad no matter what I ate.

Then, one day in 2011, someone asked me if I'd ever considered going gluten-free. I gave him a surprised look because I'd never really thought about it. I confess that my gluten knowledge was quite limited at the time. All I knew was that it was an ingredient in breads, something

I'd been eating and enjoying since I was a child. How could a simple slice of bread possibly be bad for me?

The answer is complicated, disturbing, and still shrouded in much mystery. Gluten is a protein found in wheat, barley, and rye; and it's an ingredient in a vast number of foods such as pasta, baked goods (breads, pastries, cakes, cookies, pies, etc.), cereal, pizza crust, crackers, beer, and many more. Gluten is also present in anything made with white flour, whole wheat flour, durum, semolina, kamut, spelt, triticale, and graham flour. In addition, it's used in most gravies, sauces, dressings, and marinades; and can usually be found in lunch meats, hot dogs, fried foods, soups, chips and candies. Gluten-rich foods seem to be everywhere in the normal American diet, and generations of us have grown up eating them.

The problem is that, for some unknown reason, growing numbers of people are developing varying degrees of gluten intolerance or sensitivity, meaning that the intestinal tract is unable to properly digest it. This problem can basically be divided into two distinct categories: gluten intolerance (or sensitivity) and celiac disease.

Gluten intolerance or sensitivity simply means that your body has difficulty digesting gluten. You may be able to handle various amounts of gluten on certain days, but too much may greatly increase the aforementioned symptoms and cause you to feel rather sick for a day or two. This is referred to as non-celiac gluten sensitivity, since the individual cannot tolerate gluten and demonstrates symptoms similar to someone with celiac, but does not have the antibodies and intestinal damage as seen in true celiac cases. Non-celiac gluten sensitivity is increasing at an alarming rate, and according to celiaccentral.org, 18 million Americans are currently suffering from this condition.

As for Celiac disease, it is an autoimmune disorder wherein the consumption of gluten causes visible damage to the millions of villi (tiny, tongue-like projections) in the lining of the intestines, and thus makes the sufferer unable to properly absorb vital nutrients. The damage to the villi increases permeability in the lining of the intestines, allowing toxins, bacteria, and food particles to leak through the intestinal wall and into the bloodstream. Over time, Celiac leads to pronounced malnourishment and can be fatal. A person with Celiac disease must follow a strict, life-long, gluten-free diet in order to avoid or limit serious health consequences.

A 2010 study listed by the National Institutes of Health reported that celiac disease increased five-fold over a fifteen-year period, and that the increase was due to a rapidly growing number of people losing their immunological tolerance to gluten in adulthood. The reason for this loss and the cause of celiac remain unknown.

There are many symptomatic similarities between Celiac disease and non-celiac gluten sensitivity, and the two are obviously closely related. Both can typically – but not always – produce distention and bloating of the stomach, cramping, intestinal gas, diarrhea, constipation, depression, and fatigue. The difference between the two is that Celiac can cause much more extensive damage to the intestinal wall, and lead to a wide array of dangerous health issues including type I diabetes, hypothyroidism, iron deficiency anemia, early onset osteoporosis, nervous system disorders, gallbladder malfunction, rheumatoid arthritis, and many others.

There is a battery of five blood tests typically used to check for Celiac disease. While they may not always be one hundred percent accurate (there may be false positives or negatives), these blood tests can often be reliable indicators of the presence of gluten antibodies. A biopsy of the intestinal wall is usually performed via endoscopy to confirm Celiac disease.

There are no tests to diagnose gluten intolerance. It's something that can usually be identified by eliminating gluten from your diet for a few weeks, and monitoring how your body responds. The good news is that, so far, evidence does not indicate that gluten sensitivity will necessarily lead to Celiac disease in an individual.

In either case – gluten sensitivity or Celiac disease – symptoms can usually be eliminated or greatly controlled by carefully adjusting your diet. When you stop eating foods containing gluten, your small intestine will gradually begin to heal over time, your symptoms will diminish, and your overall health should improve.

I am living proof that it can be done. Certainly, I'm often tempted by many of my favorite foods – a cheeseburger with the works, pizza, lasagna, snack crackers, chocolate chip cookies – and I do sometimes allow myself to indulge. But I know my body and my limits, and I do my best to keep a tight rein on what I eat.

Of course, it helps that more and more restaurants and grocery stores are now offering an ever-growing number of gluten-free food options. (They may not always taste quite like the "real thing," but many of them are actually very good.) Every time I go grocery shopping, it seems as though they've added another entirely new gluten-free section or aisle to the store. In fact, the gluten-free food and beverage market grew by 30 percent from 2006-2010!

As long as I maintain a daily diet that is mostly gluten-free, my symptoms are greatly reduced. The rash on my torso is gone, my bowels function much more smoothly, my abdominal distress is reduced, and I generally feel better. Believe me, if I can do it, you can do it too. It's up to you to take charge of your life and healing.

Chapter 23

Now is Wow!

Time is your enemy; time is your friend,
And this moment is infinitely coming to an end;
Time has the power to wound as it heals,
It gives as it steals from your life;
So learn to wander; learn to embrace
The lines of age upon your face;
Learn to cherish the glory and grace
Of every sweet moment you taste.

The only real power that any of us possess is the ability to choose what we will do in and with this one single moment. All we control is how we will think, feel and act in this instant. We have nothing else. We can do nothing else. There is nothing else.

The past and the future don't really exist...they're just fascinating concepts. Whatever is happening in your life is happening *right now*, not yesterday and not tomorrow. So get on board with it, no matter what it is. Don't fight or resist it. Time is marching on; get in step. The world is turning; turn with it. The entire grand experience of

Life is taking off right now; hold on tight and blast off with it.

No matter what cards you've been dealt, the time to play your hand is now. Even if you feel that you've been given the worst cards in the deck, smile and play them anyway. Engage in the game, because it's the only game in town. You're already a player whether you like it or not, and you have to do *something* with those cards. So why not choose to enjoy the game, play your hand, and make the most of it?

Even if this is the worst day, the worst moment of your entire life, it's still all you've got. Maybe you're having a panic attack like no other. Maybe your gut is in an uproar, you're sick at your stomach, and you have diarrhea from IBS. Maybe fibromyalgia is wracking your body from head to toe, and you're too weak to even crawl across the room. Or it could be that you're lying in a hospital bed, staring up at a blank ceiling, wondering if you're going to live or die. No matter what your challenge, you must choose to embrace it, right here and right now. You must choose to say 'Yes' to the moment, put a smile on your face, and empower yourself.

Therein is the key to successfully dealing with anxiety and all of the mystery diseases: how you think about things makes all the difference. And how you think about things is *entirely up to you.* It's your choice. Don't grumble about your lot in life; that accomplishes absolutely nothing. Choose not to utter a single negative word. Don't waste your time regretting your mistakes and thinking about what could have been if this or that had happened. None of that amounts to a hill of beans. You must decide that you're going to embrace the here and now with every single drop of enthusiasm and every ounce of strength you've got. Your thoughts and attitude – not your doctors and pills – are your greatest weapons in your battle against your mystery diseases.

But admittedly, all of this is much easier said than done. No one knows that better than me. I spent years thinking about the past, projecting into the future, and ignoring the Now. Much of the time, I was angry and bitter that my health had been taken from me. I held my own never-ending pity party where I regretted my mistakes, missed people who were no longer in my life, and longed for places and things I once knew and loved. And when I wasn't doing that, I spent the rest of my time and energy projecting into the future with anticipation or dread, hope or fear. *What's going to happen tomorrow, next week, or next year? How will I handle it? What will I do if this happens or that happens?* Questions like these can drive you insane and forever rob you of the here and now.

Living in the Now requires us to focus all of our energy into the present moment only, even if the moment is difficult or painful. When we're hurting or scared, we desperately want to escape the situation. That's when we long for something, anything – whether it's a drug, an injection, marijuana, alcohol, or whatever – to numb us and insulate us from the pain. The last thing we want to do is dive into the middle of it, eyes open and fully aware. We'd much rather run the opposite direction.

But that's when we must make a conscious decision to concentrate fully on what's happening in that very moment. For me, it's as if there is a little switch inside me that must be flipped to the ON position. But the switch can be very difficult to locate because it's often hidden deep within the mystery disease itself. And even when you finally find it and turn it on, sometimes it still reverts to the OFF position, again and again. You must be diligent, persistent and faithful. Just keep flipping that switch back on, and eventually it will stay on, and you'll find yourself growing spiritually as you learn to embrace the moment.

There is a glorious bliss that comes only when you learn to sit calmly in the middle of your pain. Once you can do that, you will discover depths to your spirit and being that you never dreamed existed. This is the way of wisdom, the deeper journey, the higher calling. Tears of pure joy will flow and you will feel as though you are looking into the face of God. This is an ecstasy that cannot be adequately described and cannot be surpassed. You will understand only when you experience it, when it rolls over you like waves of peace on the Sea of Now.

We grow in the meditative slivers of silence,
And the prayerful seasons of sorrow;
When root and bloom become One,
We burst forth in the glory of the grand moment.

Chapter 24

Tasty Tidbits

Right now, decide that you are going to be the most loving and wonderful person in the entire world.

Stress less, soar more.

Speak no evil, for words are far more powerful than we ever imagined. You cannot spew verbal filth and negativism from your mouth and remain unaffected by it.

Giving is living. This is a novel concept in our I-Me-Mine society.

Time spent in a hospital bed *as* a patient helps you *become* more patient.

Some days require pure grit; other days, whispered prayers.

Some days are bathed in smiles, while others are washed in tears.

Complaint will taint the soul, but praise will raise the spirit.

Determine that mediocrity is not good enough. Strive for greatness.

Meditation *will* improve your life.

There are some things – and people – you just can't fix, no matter how hard you try.

You are not the judge or the jury.

Choose to forgive those who have hurt you. This may be the most difficult thing in the world, but do it anyway. And while you're at it, pray for your enemies and those who spitefully use and abuse you.

Optimism, confidence and determination are formidable foes. Keep them on your side.

Exercise caution when it comes to the wonders and complexities of your brain, neurochemicals, and hormones. Consider the very real possibility that your answers are not always found in a pill bottle or a syringe.

Don't reinforce negative storylines in your own life or in the world at large.

Eliminate all regrets about the past, and cease all worries about the unknown variables of the future.

Sometimes we look around and complain, and wish things could be better. But wishing is like fishing without a pole. Put your wishes to work.

Sometimes we find God in the crisis, in the crucible of sorrow or horror; and occasionally He comes in the form of a burning bush, earthquake, or the deafening roar of thunder. But we can also find God in the everyday things, hidden in the ordinary, and in the silence when and where we least expect Him.

Fearful "What-if?" thinking only feeds anxiety and panic; stop it now!

When you come to the end of your rope, tie it around your ankle and dangle upside down for a while. You'll see everything from a new perspective.

You can never go wrong by doing right.

Change the way you think, change your decision-making process, and it will have a powerful, positive effect on you and every aspect of your life.

If you're too busy to be nice to people, then you're too busy.

The secret is not in the answer; it's in the question.

Even if you think you're the most lopsided, screwed-up, lost soul on the planet, there's still hope for you. You have the power and potential to change your life, right here and now, one decision and one step at a time.

The past is untouchable, the future unknowable, and only the present is doable.

Approach every new day as if it's Christmas morning; rip the wrapping paper off and enjoy!

Chapter 25

Healthy Habits

Much of what I have learned about healing, living and thriving with my mystery diseases doesn't involve the outward *doing of things*. It's not about doctors, drugs, fad diets, workout routines, or the latest medical techniques. It's about the Spirit, the inner man, attitude and the way you think. It's about the will to live and the desire to move forward. Most importantly, it's about the true juggernauts that reside within you: faith, hope and love. To unleash them, I recommend you employ the following healthy habits.

BE THE BOSS

You must take charge of your healing and your life because no one knows your body, mind and needs better than you do. Though medical science can do amazing things, there is still much they do not yet understand about the complexities of the human body and mind. Therefore, you must not allow doctors, nurses, drugs, friends, family, or even your own pain to rule you. You must exercise your innate right to control your own treatment plan and make decisions that are best for you.

MEDITATE

Stress, worry, and pain are powerful forces, and they can only be effectively managed or conquered by exercising the power of your mind, will and focused intention. Mind-body techniques such as meditation, combined with controlled breathing and a powerful mantra, will balance and strengthen your immune system, allowing you to fight off illness, rest better, and heal more quickly.

You must set aside a time each day for this vital practice, and stick to it. *Meditation has been my greatest tool in the process of overcoming my mystery diseases.* Read that sentence again. I can state unequivocally that meditation is by far the most powerful instrument in the process of learning how to calm, center, ground, and heal oneself. It allows you to tap into the boundless wonder of the universe, and enables you to finally and fully understand that you are nothing more or less than a single, glorious lightning bolt flashing across the vast sky. And with that realization, you will be more free and powerful than you ever imagined.

RETRAIN YOUR BRAIN

We've all seen those Clearance Sale commercials where an announcer proclaims, "Everything must go!" That is exactly the approach you must take in order to begin the retraining process. Consciously and repeatedly release and discard all bitterness, self-doubt, self-pity, and anger. Throw out absolutely every piece of negativity that resides anywhere in your head. Then, fill your brain with only positive, productive, and life-affirming ways of living and thinking. You must be judicious and tenacious in this process. Out with the old, in with the new; out with the false, in with the true.

CHOOSE WISELY

We all make thousands of decisions and choices every day. Eggs or cereal for breakfast? The blue shirt or the maroon one? Do these pants make my rear end look big? Fill up with gas now or hold off till later? Park here or hope for a better space closer to the door? Where are we going for lunch? Should I take this job offer or stay where I am? Get married now or wait? Interstate or back road? Burial or cremation? Facebook or Twitter? Paper or plastic? Coke or Pepsi? Do you want fries with that?

No one can make all these decisions for you, but there are several choices I highly recommend and urge you to make: *Choose to say 'Yes' to this moment, no matter what it holds. Choose to smile no matter how much you hurt. Choose to be filled with gratitude for all the good things in the Universe and in your life. Choose to show love no matter how others treat you. Choose to be the very best person you can possibly be.* If you first make these wise choices, you will be grounded on a firm foundation. Then all your other decisions will be birthed in wisdom and fall neatly into place.

BE ACTIVE

For people with fibromyalgia, chronic pain or chronic fatigue, it can be very difficult to exercise; but it's important that you keep moving and stay busy even when you don't feel your best. Know your limits, but do as much as you can. Don't worry about meeting anyone else's expectations, and don't fret about what you used to be able to do before your mystery disease came along. Just learn to ride the waves of your illness, reach deep down inside, and give it all you've got. Walk while you're on the phone. Stretch while you watch TV. Dance when you listen to music. Do jumping jacks while you're driving. Okay, maybe not that last one.

EAT WELL

Enjoy your food, but bear in mind that its main purpose is to serve as sustenance. Food isn't something to be worshipped and obsessed over; it's primarily fuel that your body needs to operate at maximum efficiency. Don't chase after the endless stream of fad diets and gimmicks. Just make certain that you consistently eat in a healthy manner by consuming a wide variety of foods that are packed with vitamins, minerals, antioxidants, and fiber. Eat plenty of almonds, dark green vegetables, red beans, fresh fruits, and broiled fish. Make these items the staples of your diet, and then build from there.

For people with IBS, gluten sensitivity, lactose intolerance, or other gastrointestinal problems, eating well is an even greater challenge. But it can be done by keeping a detailed food journal and learning how your body and digestive system respond to various foods. Discover which foods or ingredients trigger your gastro-intestinal flare-ups, and be sure to avoid those things. It's okay to relish the many succulent flavors and diverse food tastes that the world has to offer, but remember to do all things in moderation. And unless you have severe allergies or reactions to certain foods, it can even be okay to "cheat" a little bit from time to time, as long as you do it carefully and moderately.

I often think of the advice given by my great uncle Sid who lived to be more than 100 years old. When interviewed by local media on his ninetieth birthday, he was asked to explain the secret of such a long and remarkably healthy life. With a twinkle in his eye, he said, "Never skip dessert."

DOCTOR UP

Yes, I have made it abundantly clear that you must take charge of your own healing, but that does not necessarily exclude having a good doctor. And though you may have been disappointed in the past by members of the medical community, there are still some great health care professionals out there. You simply have to find one who is intelligent, open-minded, and with whom you feel comfortable. Doctors certainly don't have all the answers, but they do have a wealth of knowledge, training and experience. Find one you trust and allow him or her to assist you and walk with you on your journey to better health.

INTERACT

You'll be amazed at how much better you'll feel if you reconnect with old friends, make new ones, and have activities to look forward to. Plus, the more you keep yourself occupied, the less time you have to feel bad or to sit around feeling sorry for yourself. Join a club, organization, church group, or sports team. Take a night class, or teach one, for that matter. You'll feel better if you interact with other people. Listen, learn and love.

PUSH YOURSELF

Get outside your comfort zone, and stretch your boundaries in every possible direction. You're an atheist? Attend church. Hate sports? Join a softball league. You're right-handed? Start doing things with your left hand. Love the Yankees? Wear a Red Sox cap. Love money? Give some away to a stranger.

HAVE FUN

Don't be afraid to act silly sometimes, because it can be very therapeutic. Buy some crayons and a children's coloring book; then spread them out on the floor and color like a kid. Take a bubble bath and play with a toy boat.

Watch a few of the old Looney Tunes cartoons and allow yourself a bushel of belly-laughs. Blow bubbles outside in the sunlight. Wiggle your toes in the grass. Put on some classic, bubblegum pop music like The Partridge Family or The Osmonds, and sing along! Do whatever it takes to regain that childlike wonder and joy for living.

LOVE

Love yourself. Love your family and friends. Love the unlovable. Rescue an animal from a shelter, and take it into your home and your heart. Buy or grow some plants and tend to them gently. Begin to notice and love the little things in life that may have once seemed so insignificant. It may sound cliché or foolish to you, but I encourage you to literally hug a tree and smell the roses. Whisper to them and thank them for being a part of this big, beautiful world.

No, I haven't lost my mind; I found it, actually. And now I understand that even if every muscle in your body is aching, even if your heart is breaking, even if you think you've reached the end of your rope; smile and embrace every single, glorious moment of your journey. Love God, love the Universe, love Life, love the Earth, love yourself, and love others with every last ounce of strength you possess.

Chapter 26

Appetizing Axioms

When you have a million and one things to do, start with the one.

If you're going through hell, drink plenty of water.

The only thing you will ever gain from worry is the realization that worry gains you nothing.

Stop the wondering why and focus on the healing how.

Medical science, technology, statistics and double-blind studies are wonderful, but they are not the be-all and end-all of understanding the health of a human being. You can't put a life in a test tube.

No one really wants to die; but, on the bright side, it will effectively get you out of dinner with your in-laws.

Recognize the beauty in change; don't resist it. Simply see yourself as moving from one beautiful part of your life to the next.

You can't have grace under fire without a fire.

Whining and complaining are equally effective strategies for healing. Neither one works.

If making money is more important to you than making someone happy, then you are making a big mistake.

According to statistics, statistics never lie.

Choose your friends wisely. Avoid insensitive and negative people who steal your joy, prey on your tenderness, and drain your strength.

Just when you think you've reached a higher state of enlightenment, Windows comes out with a new version.

Find a purpose for your life that is larger than your losses.

You are a physical, mental, emotional and spiritual being; what affects one of these aspects of you, affects ALL of them.

Learn to see your enemies as teachers, not as foes; and thank them for the lessons they've taught you.

The secret to life, joy and peace is to say 'Yes' to life, just as it is presented to you, not just when it bends to your wishes, because it rarely will.

In baseball, it's always exciting to see a batter stretch a single into a double. Life is a lot like baseball.

Holding a grudge is like trying to hold onto an angry cat.

It's easy to be bitter, and cynicism is a piece of cake; but daily walking the high road of faith, hope and love is where the challenge and reward are found.

You will most certainly fail every time you do not try.

Realize that, even as brilliant as you may think you are, there is much you do not know. Make friends with people who hold differing opinions from yours on politics, religion and laundry detergent. Then listen and learn.

Remember the Titanic. Always have an oar and a bucket handy.

It's natural to prefer the easy path, but it's hard to be great without great obstacles.

The box is not your friend.

Relish is life's most important condiment. Never leave home without it!

It's foolish to deny your pain, for there is no healing without hurting.

In spite of all our human faults and weaknesses, we are glorious creatures, capable of boundless creativity, unrivaled ingenuity, and marvelous wonders of love and compassion.

Chapter 27

The Good News

Since 1995 I have lived with my ever-expanding list of mystery diseases: anxiety disorders, panic attacks, intestinal bleeding, agoraphobia, depression, chronic fatigue syndrome, gluten sensitivity, lactose intolerance, irritable bowel syndrome, alcoholism, restless leg syndrome, obsessive compulsive disorder, manic episodes, fibromyalgia, eating disorders, and many more.

I experience so many radical mood changes and energy swings that I could probably be the poster boy for mood disorders! Some days I hurt so badly that I can't get out of bed and I feel like I'm 95 years old. Other days I have an incredible burst of energy, my symptoms recede a bit, and I soar through the stratosphere of life. But most days I'm somewhere in between those two, fighting the good fight, keeping the faith.

Some people have called me a fool for battling my health problems without an armload of pharmaceutical products. Maybe I am. But for 18 years I have, for the most part, faced my demons and mystery diseases head on, without having my senses dulled, my personality changed, or my enthusiasm dampened by drugs. Life is a long road, however, and I have enough wisdom to realize that, as I age, medications may become necessary. But for now, I plan to stay the course.

I am not saying this is the path for everyone to follow – I judge no one – but it has been the path for me. I've often put myself, by choice, in the thick of the battle with no buffer, no medications to insulate me. At times it's been beyond glorious, and at times terrifying; but I've fought the battle mostly on my terms, and I do not regret a moment of it.

I want to make it abundantly clear that I have great admiration for the tremendous accomplishments of medical science. And I want to make it equally clear that, in many cases, medications are necessary and effective for healing and curing various diseases. I am not suggesting that anyone who takes prescription drugs is somehow weak or inferior. Some illnesses are diagnosed rather easily and quickly, and can be effectively treated with medications. But many diseases fall into the mystery category; they cannot be easily diagnosed, and there is no clear or useful pharmaceutical treatment method. It is these cases, the mystery diseases, to which I refer; and each individual must decide for himself how best to deal with his affliction.

In fact, this is one of the most important lessons I've learned along the way: *Your health and healing are largely up to you, the patient.* There are many bright, well-intentioned doctors, nurses and support staff in the health-care field who truly care about you, but they can only do so much. And your family and friends can give love, assistance and support, but they can never fully understand or "fix" what you're going through. Ultimately, at the end of the day, you are the greatest advocate for your health and well-being. You must take charge and steer the ship, because no one knows your body, mind, and needs better than you.

I also learned to seek God's help and wisdom. It's a way of humbling yourself before the Creator and the Creation, admitting that you don't know everything, and opening yourself up to the unknown and unlimited possibilities that the Universe may hold for you. Human beings are complex and amazing creatures, indeed, but there is a lot to be said for putting your faith in something much bigger than yourself. Sometimes you have to drop your preconceived agenda, open your mind, and be willing to listen, learn and grow.

For years I watched my health deteriorate, and I was angry and bitter about what my mysterious diseases were doing to me. But over time, I faced my fears, worked through the pain, and came to see my afflictions as a blessing. I won't even pretend to tell you that it's been easy, or that I don't still have my share of bad moments. Sometimes I still grumble, lose my calm demeanor, or whine about my problems. I'm still very much a work in progress, and I have a long way to go.

But have I changed? How could I not?! More than ever before, I believe in myself, trust in others, and have faith in God. I am learning to find hope in hopeless situations, show compassion when hearts are hard, trust that love will win out, and tremble with joy over even the smallest things. And the strangest mystery of all: the deeper my sorrow, the greater my gratitude. Mine is most certainly not a tale of sadness; it is my story of *choosing to smile in the midst of sadness.*

I believe our society is being overwhelmed by a rising, raging sea of neurological disorders, immune-related diseases, mood disturbance disorders, and life-threatening gastrointestinal problems. So far, a hundred million of our citizens are battling the strange symptoms of this 21st century crop of mystery diseases. But no one knows exactly why, and the answer is most certainly incredibly complex and multi-layered.

Who can yet say what we are doing to ourselves with our rapidly evolving society, shifting of cultural structures, technological whirlwinds, and massive quantities of unbridled stress? How and when will we know what damage we've done by pumping ourselves full of chemicals, preservatives, genetically-modified foods, radiation, electromagnetic fields, processed sugar, water contaminants and air pollution?

The evidence is indisputable: we have saturated our soil, water and air with man-made chemicals and substances. How could we possibly avoid ingesting them into our lungs, mouths, and the pores of our skin? And it may be that we are just now seeing the tip of the iceberg. If that sounds extreme or alarmist, so be it. Perhaps I am singing like a canary in a coal mine in days of yore. But I'm not the only one.

Regardless, healing can still begin today inside of you and me. Take charge of your journey. Follow the simple steps I outlined in the previous chapter. Change your life and the world too. Eat well, have fun and laugh a lot. Soak in the sunlight. Do only those things that will keep your conscience clear, and then sleep peacefully at night. Love everybody, and give extra attention to the special people in your life. Slow down, temper your workaholic ways, begin a daily meditation practice, and slip off those shackles put on you by our dollar-first, win-at-all-costs, western society.

I was once firmly entrenched in that lifestyle, and I was bitter about how things turned out. I complained and whined far too often. *Why God? Why do these things always happen to me? Why do I have to be sick? Why can't I catch a break? Why does everybody else have all the good luck? Why did you do this to me?* And after years of asking such foolish and destructive questions, I fell into the abyss.

145

I will not sugarcoat the truth: pain is no picnic, and suffering is not for sissies. But pain and suffering teach us how to endure and make us stronger. And that, in turn, builds character. And then, surprisingly, mysteriously, and gloriously, we discover hope, joy and peace. Right at the place where we least expected, we find them. The process isn't easy, but it is most definitely worth it. Your disease – mystery or otherwise – is not a curse; it's your greatest blessing, *if you choose it to be so*. It's not destroying you; it's giving you the opportunity to soar.

Realize that every part and parcel of our existence – all our frailties and fears, all our comforts and conquests – are vital components of our human journey on Planet Earth. These are the ingredients that cause us to sizzle in the beautiful skillet of life.

And even now as I sit here writing this final chapter, with one of my favorite prayer candles burning, I slip in and out of prose and prayer, musing and meditating. I stare into the perfect flame and I can see myself as a little boy, opening that cellar door and stepping into the unknown darkness. I close my eyes and suddenly I'm a young father, laughing and romping in the floor with three precious children. Then the years scroll by and I have become a successful businessman, chasing the almighty dollar, working too hard and drinking too much. Finally, I see myself in a hospital bed, staring up at a blank ceiling, contemplating ways to end my life.

The Earth turns and night becomes day, and the sun smiles with the most beautiful ray. Pain and fear have been my teachers, and the journey of learning is the glorious reward, worth every sorrow and loss. I've come full circle with tears of joy streaming down my face, and a song of hope in my heart that no mystery disease can ever silence.

Chapter 28

Magnificent Morsels

Always choose the high road. There are fewer potholes and a better view.

It's hard to be great without great challenges.

Everybody likes doughnuts. Be the doughnut in someone's life.

Don't resist truth, because if you run from the light long enough, sooner or later it's going to get very dark.

It takes great strength to embrace your weaknesses, and true courage to embrace your fear.

An epiphany shines like a beacon from the mountaintop, urging you there.

The path to wisdom can be long and arduous, so be sure to wear comfortable shoes.

We all have skeletons in our closet. Some of us need a bigger closet.

To keep your heart pure, you must keep it out of the dirt.

Your illness or circumstances may rob you of many things, but they cannot take away your determination or dignity, your faith or joy, unless you allow them.

Success in business is 50% determination, 50% hard work, and 50% math skills.

For success in life, attitude is everything. Hard work is also everything.

Sometimes we have a right to be angry, but we don't have a right to be cruel.

You can't learn from the mistakes you refuse to acknowledge.

Dreams are the wings upon which we soar.

The power of suggestion is very real, and the human mind is a super-charged suggestion box. So fill it with good ideas, not bad ones.

Think well, for action follows thought.

Only a tennis player likes a back-handed compliment.

Pain and pleasure, joy and sorrow, are simply opposite sides of the same very thin coin.

When you are hurting, sick or dying, having someone at your side who truly loves you is worth more than all the money in the world.

A closed mind is an open door to ignorance and fear.

Sometimes when you follow the crowd, you walk right off a cliff.

Love trumps the combined might of all the traditions, ceremonies, labels, classifications, rules, rituals, procedures, prestige, possessions, and money in the world. And it's not even close.

When you resist what is, you are like water trying not to be wet.

Mistakes are little books that make us wise, if we read them carefully.

Stop worrying about all the things you think you can't be, and focus on the one thing you *can* be – YOU.

Love like you breathe.

Every day, you are given a blank canvas and a big box of crayons. Why not create something beautiful?

The next time someone tells you that something can't be done, remind them that most of mankind's greatest accomplishments were once considered impossible.

Live each day with a fiery, insatiable curiosity. Never stop reaching out, reaching forward, reaching up to your highest potential.

Faith is greater than fear, and love is stronger than death.

Human

I've been a lover, a fighter, a winner and a loser
A joker, a jerk, and once even a boozer
I've been a lone wolf, and I've run with the pack
Been so far gone I thought I'd never get back

Been put off, put down, put up on a pedestal
Over-worked, unemployed, needing major medical
I've been a fool for love, and sometimes just a fool
And though I fall short, I still believe in the Golden Rule

> So with childlike faith I will walk in wonder
> Until they put me six feet under
> All I can do is do my best
> Nothing more and nothing less
> I'm not perfect, I confess….
> I'm just human

I've knocked down some walls and mended fences
Stood with my friends side by side in the trenches
I've seen real beauty and it's more than skin-deep
It's the love you give away, and the promises you keep

My straight and narrow has been a crooked path
I've been wounded and weary but I can still laugh
I'm a work in progress, learning patience today
What will the Master make from this lump of clay?

With childlike faith I will walk in wonder
Until they put me six feet under
All I can do is do my best
In spite of my recklessness
I'm not perfect, I freely confess….
I'm just human

I'm not making excuses
For who I am or the things that I've done
I've still got a long way to go
But just look at how far I have come…

I'm a child, a parent, a friend, a foe
A unique individual, an average Joe
Over-achieving, underrated, full of hope, somewhat jaded
Pampered and bruised, clear-headed and confused
So please try to understand…
I'm just human

And with childlike faith I will walk in wonder
Until they put me six feet under
All I can do is do my best
Nothing more and nothing less
I'm not perfect, I confess….
I'm just human

Appendix

This section provides an alphabetical listing and a brief definition of a wide variety of mysterious, unusual and fascinating diseases and disorders; followed by examples of well-known individuals who have been diagnosed with or were widely considered to have had each condition.

Acquired Immune Deficiency Syndrome (AIDS): AIDS is a condition that develops when a body has been weakened by the human immunodeficiency virus (HIV). HIV damages the immune system so that the body is no longer able to fight off common germs and pathogens. HIV can be spread by sharing needles in drug use or through unprotected sex.
Actor Rock Hudson, singer Freddie Mercury, tennis star Arthur Ashe, author Isaac Asimov, basketball star Magic Johnson, Olympic diver Greg Louganis, AIDS activist Elizabeth Glaser.

Addison's Disease: chronic adrenal deficiency caused by the gradual destruction of the adrenal glands by the body's immune system. Addison's is also referred to as primary adrenal insufficiency and can be life-threatening.
President John F. Kennedy, author Jane Austen, singer Helen Reddy.

Agoraphobia: fear of being outside of one's home or in a crowded area.

Television chef Paula Deen, tennis star Andre Agassi, scientist Charles Darwin, actor Billy Bob Thornton, actress/sex symbol Marilyn Monroe, filmmaker Woody Allen.

Alzheimer's Disease: a degenerative brain disorder and the most common form of dementia. The cause of Alzheimer's is unknown and there is no effective treatment. It is the sixth leading cause of death in the United States.
Senator Barry Goldwater, actress Rita Hayworth, singer Perry Como, boxer Sugar Ray Robinson, actor Charlton Heston, President Ronald Reagan.

Amyotrophic Lateral Sclerosis (ALS): neurological disease that causes progressive muscle weakness, disability and eventually death. Also known as Lou Gehrig's Disease for the famous New York Yankees baseball player.
Actor David Niven, Chinese leader Mao Zedong, baseball player James "Catfish" Hunter, physicist/author Stephen Hawking.

Anisakiasis: a zoonotic disease that can occur when a person ingests larval nematodes (worms) present in raw fish and other raw seafood dishes. The worms cause nausea, vomiting and other symptoms; and can sometimes become invasive and migrate to other parts of the body.

Anorexia: an eating disorder characterized by a markedly reduced appetite or a total aversion to food.
Singer Karen Carpenter, singer Fiona Apple, actress Calista Flockheart, actress Tara Reid, actress Mary Kate Olsen, models Shane and Sia Barbi (The Barbi Twins).

Anxiety Disorder: a chronic condition of excessive worry and severe apprehension causing a wide range of uncomfortable and disturbing symptoms.
Singer John Mayer, singer George Michael, inventor Nikolas Tesla, poet Emily Dickinson, weatherman Willard Scott, scientist Sigmund Freud.

Aquagenic Urticaria: a rare disorder that causes itchy, burning, or painful red or white lumps, rash or hives on a person's skin after contact with water. The cause is unknown and the disease may affect only portions or the entire body. It can occur after bathing, swimming, or merely walking in the rain; and the temperature of the water has no bearing on the symptoms. Also known as water allergy.

Aseptic Meningitis: serous inflammation of the linings of the brain that causes headache, fever, nausea and other symptoms. It is similar to viral meningitis and it can be difficult to distinguish between the two. Aseptic meningitis is often benign but can be fatal.

Asperger Syndrome (AS): an autism spectrum disorder (ASD) characterized by impairment of social skills, poor communication abilities, and repetitive behavior patterns.
Pokeman creator Satoshi Tajiri, actress Daryl Hannah, author Dawn Prince-Hughes Ph.D.

Asthma: a chronic lung disease that inflames and narrows the air passageways, and causes wheezing, shortness of breath, chest tightness, and coughing. While the exact cause of asthma is unknown, and there is no cure; symptoms can usually be managed with medicines, proper lifestyle management, and avoidance techniques.
Politician Rev. Jesse Jackson, Olympic athlete Jackie Joyner-Kersee, President Calvin Coolidge, singer Alice

Cooper, President Bill Clinton, director Martin Scorsese, publisher/philanthropist Joseph Pulitzer, football star Emmitt Smith.

Ataxophobia: fear of disorder or untidiness. This is often considered to be the opposite of a hoarder.
Soccer star David Beckham.

Attention Deficit Hyperactivity Disorder (ADHD): a wide range of problematic behaviors such as persistent inattention, hyperactivity, impulsivity, and restlessness that interfere with interpersonal relationships and employment. Also referred to as Attention Deficit Disorder (ADD).
Singer/actor Justin Timberlake, Olympic swimmer Michael Phelps, actor/comedian Jim Carrey, television personality Ty Pennington, professional football star/TV personality Terry Bradshaw, model/TV personality Paris Hilton.

Autism: a serious developmental problem that usually appears before age 3, and seems to be sharply on the rise in recent decades. It typically causes problems in social interaction, language and behavior, though it can vary widely from person to person.
Author/linguist Daniel Tammet, author/professor Temple Grandin Ph.D.

Avian Flu: a bird flu that can sometimes be transmitted to humans by contact with bird droppings. In addition to typical flu-like symptoms, Avian Flu can also attack the respiratory system, brain, or digestive tract. It is often fatal.

Bell's Palsy: a neurological disorder that causes the sudden onset of facial paralysis resulting from decreased blood flow or compression of cranial nerves. The exact cause of Bell's Palsy is unknown.
Singer Carnie Wilson, actress/comedian Roseanne Barr, actor George Clooney, politician/activist Ralph Nader, composer Sir Andrew Lloyd Webber.

Benign Fasciculation Syndrome (BFS): unexplained and continuous muscle twitching, tremor, and cramping throughout the body.

Bipolar Disorder: drastic mood swings from lows of depression to highs of mania. Also referred to as manic-depressive disorder.
Actor Mel Gibson, singer Kurt Cobain, singer Ozzy Osbourne, artist Vincent van Gogh, actress Vivien Leigh, actress/author Carrie Fisher.

Bow Hunter's Stroke: a rare type of stroke caused by obstruction or narrowing of the main arteries supplying blood to the brainstem or cerebellum. In some individuals it may be caused by forcibly turning one's head from side to side, which can impair blood flow in the upper neck where the arteries enter the brain. This condition was first identified in 1978 by Dr. B.F. Sorenson in his patient who was an archer and frequent bow hunter.

Bulimia: an eating disorder characterized by episodes of secretive, excessive binge-eating, followed by self-induced vomiting, abuse of laxatives, or excessive exercise.
Actor/comedian Russell Brand, actress Lindsay Lohan, singer/TV personality Paula Abdul, actress Jane Fonda, Princess Diana, singer Elton John, singer Alanis Morissette, comedian Joan Rivers, actress Jamie-Lynn

Sigler, singer Britney Spears, singer Amy Winehouse, exercise guru Richard Simmons.

Candidiasis: an infection caused by the fungus *Candidas Albicans* that can infect the mouth, skin, vagina, or urinary tract. Invasive candidiasis occurs when the fungus enters the bloodstream; it is the fourth most common bloodstream infection among hospitalized patients in the United States.

Celiac Disease: an autoimmune disease wherein the consumption of gluten initiates damage to the lining of the intestines, and makes one unable to properly absorb nutrients. Over time, Celiac leads to malnourishment and can be fatal.
Historian/author Sarah Vowell, sports/TV personality Keith Olbermann, TV personality Elisabeth Hasselback, professional football star Drew Brees.

Chronic Fatigue Syndrome (CFS): extreme and inexplicable fatigue that does not improve with rest. Sufferers may be bedridden for days at a time.
Move director Blake Edwards, soccer star Michelle Akers, singer Stevie Nicks, singer/actress Cher, motocross racer Ricky Carmichael, writer/publicist Howard Bloom.

Common Cold: this sickness typically lasts a few days and causes runny nose, stuffy nose, itchy throat, sneezing, coughing, some body ache, and mild fatigue. Medical science still doesn't fully understand this illness, and cannot prevent it or cure it.
Almost everyone on the planet.

Complex Regional Pain Syndrome (CRPS): a chronic pain condition resulting from a malfunction of the nervous system. The pain is progressive, usually affects one of the limbs, and may cause dramatic changes in skin color, temperature and swelling of the affected area. Formerly known as Reflex Sympathetic Dystrophy. *Singer/TV personality Paula Abdul.*

Conn's Syndrome: a very rare disorder that occurs when the adrenal glands produce too much aldosterone, a hormone that controls sodium and potassium levels in the blood. This overproduction causes retention of salt and a loss of potassium, which leads to hypertension. Conn's may present with high blood pressure, headaches, muscle cramps and weakness, excessive thirst and urination, and heart problems. Conn's is typically curable.

Cotard's Syndrome: a strange psychiatric disorder wherein the patient is convinced that he has lost his organs, blood, or soul; or has died or become a zombie. Also referred to as Walking Corpse Syndrome.

Coulrophobia: fear of clowns.
Actor Johnny Depp, rapper P. Diddy, comedian Carol Burnett.

Creutzfeldt-Jakob Disease (CJD): a rare and mysterious neurodegenerative disorder that progresses rapidly and is always fatal. The cause is not known and may be the result of a slow virus or another as yet unknown organism with an incubation period as long as 50 years. CJD may be related to Mad Cow Disease.
Silicon Valley executive Mike Homer.

Crohn's Disease: an autoimmune disorder which causes chronic inflammation of the gastrointestinal tract. This condition may affect any area of the GI tract and cause a wide range of distressing symptoms in various parts of the body. The cause of Crohn's remains largely a mystery, as does an effective treatment. Persistent symptoms such as intestinal bleeding often require surgery to remove a large portion of the intestines.

Television personality Frank Fritz, news correspondent Cynthia McFadden, actress Shannen Doherty, NHL hockey player/coach Kevin Dineen, singer Anastacia.

Cushing's Disease: a rare but serious hormonal disorder caused by high levels of the hormone cortisol in the body over a prolonged period of time. Excessive cortisol can be caused by either medications or a malfunction or tumor in the body's endocrine system.

Depression: a mental disorder characterized by sadness, feelings of guilt or low self-worth, disturbed appetite or sleep, loss of interest or pleasure in things, poor concentration and fatigue.

Singer Sheryl Crow, actor/comedian Jim Carrey, comedian/TV personality Drew Carey, US Senator Thomas Eagleton, astronaut Buzz Aldrin, actor Heath Ledger, author J.K. Rowling, President Teddy Roosevelt.

Diffuse Esophageal Spasm (DES): abnormal and distressing contractions of unknown origin in the esophagus which cause difficulty swallowing and pain in the chest and upper abdomen.

Eating Disorders Not Otherwise Specified (EDNOS): catch-all category of dangerous eating behaviors, such as binge eating, that do not fall into the anorexia or bulimia categories. (*see OSFED.) [Note: reclassification will designate this disorder to be given a new description of Other Specified Feeding and Eating Disorders (OSFED) as the new Diagnostic and Statistical Manual of Mental Disorders (DSM-5) replaces the old (DSM-4).]

Actress/singer Jamie-Lynn Sigler, actress/singer Nicole Richie.

Elephantitis: extreme enlargement of the arms, legs or genitals caused by parasitic round worm infection. This disease appears to be on the increase worldwide, but can sometimes be effectively treated if caught in the early stages of infection.

Epidermodysplasia Verruciformis (Tree Bark Skin Disorder): a very rare skin condition characterized by wart-like skin eruptions that may sometimes form clusters with an appearance similar to tree bark. Caused by infection with the human papillomavirus, this disease is usually, but not always, hereditary.

Epilepsy: a neurological condition of unknown origin that causes seizures. Signs of a seizure can include convulsions, eyes rolling back, temporary deafness or blindness, unconsciousness, teeth clenching, drooling and many others.
Author Truman Capote, musician Lindsay Buckingham, Olympic champion Florence Griffith Joyner, author Charles Dickens, French emperor Napoleon Bonaparte.

Erythromelalgia (EM): an often devastating disorder that causes the feet and/or hands to turn bright red or blue, and to burn with extreme pain. Sufferers are often forced to put their feet or hands in buckets of ice water in an effort to reduce the pain. Little is known about this affliction and there is no cure or relief. Also known as Mitchell's Disease or Burning Feet Syndrome.

Farmer's Lung: acute or chronic hypersensitivity pneumonitis caused by inhalation of moldy hay or compost contaminated with mold spores or fungi.

Farmer's Lung can cause a wide range of distressing symptoms including fever, chronic cough, malaise, lung disease, and death.

Fibromyalgia: chronic, wide-spread musculoskeletal pain, joint stiffness, and extreme fatigue.
Singer Sinead O'Connor, actor Michael James Hastings, comedian Janeane Garofalo, actor Morgan Freeman, nurse/social reformer Florence Nightingale.

Generalized Anxiety Disorder (GAD): excessive worry and tension for no apparent reason which causes distressing physical symptoms and impairs one's ability to function on a daily basis.
President Abraham Lincoln, singer/TV personality Donny Osmond, singer George Michael, singer Leann Rimes.

Gigantism (Acromegaly): abnormally large growth due to an excess of growth hormone produced by the pituitary gland. This is often due to a tumor on the pituitary gland, but there are also other causes.
Wrestler/actor Andre the Giant, actor Richard Kiel.

Gluten Sensitivity or Intolerance: having a negative reaction to gluten (wheat) which produces a wide variety of symptoms such as abdominal bloating, cramping, pain, gas, diarrhea, constipation, headaches, joint pain, muscle ache, depression, anxiety, eczema, acne, and fatigue.
Actress/singer Zooey Deschanel, singer Jessica Simpson, actor Billy Bob Thornton, tennis star Novak Djokovic, Olympic runner Amy Yoder Begley.

Graves' Disease: an autoimmune disorder that causes an over-production of thyroid hormones. Its bodily symptoms and effects are wide-ranging, and Graves' is the most common cause of hyperthyroidism.

Singer Toni Childs, Olympian Gail Devers, rapper Missy Elliott.

Guillain-Barre Syndrome: a disorder of the peripheral nervous system that may cause numbness, muscle weakness, paralysis, or death. It is an autoimmune disease of unknown origin that appears to follow an acute infectious process.
President Franklin D. Roosevelt, Quarterback Danny Wuerfful, author Joseph Heller, actor Andy Griffith.

Harlequin Syndrome: an odd condition in which one side of a person's body flushes and sweats, while the other side remains normal. With a clear line of demarcation between the two halves, the flushing may appear as a bright sunburn and the sweating is often excessive. Harlequin Syndrome appears to be caused by some sort of trauma to or malfunction by the sympathetic nervous system between the shoulder blades.

Hashimoto's Disease: an autoimmune disorder in which the immune system attacks the thyroid gland, causing inflammation and eventually destruction of the gland. It creates a wide range of distressing symptoms, but it can usually be controlled with medication. Hashimoto's is the most common cause of hypothyroidism.
Actress Kim Cattrall, actress Gena Lee Nolin,

Hypertrichosis (Werewolf Disease): very rare condition that causes thick groupings of hair to grow on various parts of the face and body. It may manifest as generalized (hair all over the body) or localized (hair only on specific parts of the body). Hypertrichosis is typically caused by a genetic mutation on the X chromosome
Jo-Jo the Dog-Faced Boy (Barnum & Bailey Circus), Supatra "Nat" Sasuphan (the world's hairiest child).

Ichthyosis Vulgaris (Fish Scale Disease): a disorder characterized by a buildup of thick, dry scales on one's skin. This condition is typically hereditary, but not in every case.

Inflammatory Bowel Disease (IBD): chronic and life-threatening inflammation of the digestive tract. IBD includes diseases such as Crohn's and ulcerative colitis.
Football player David Garrard, actress Shannen Doherty, professional wrestler George 'The Animal' Steele, President Dwight D. Eisenhower.

Insomnia: chronic inability to fall asleep or remain asleep for an adequate amount of time.
Singer Elvis Presley, painter Vincent Van Gogh, actress Judy Garland, President Abraham Lincoln.

Irritable Bowel Syndrome (IBS): disorder that affects the large intestine (colon), causing abdominal pain and cramping, changes in bowel movements, mucus in stools, diarrhea and constipation.
Model/TV personality Tyra Banks, rapper Cam 'Ron, TV star Chyler Leigh, actress Cybill Shepherd, baseball player Franklin Gutierrez, rock star Kurt Cobain, President John F. Kennedy.

Jamaican Vomiting Sickness (JVS): a mysterious disease once considered to be linked primarily to malnutrition or psychogenic causes. While much remains unknown about this sickness, it appears to be an often fatal reaction to consuming unripe ackee fruit. JVS can cause a variety of distressing symptoms including extreme vomiting, convulsions, and death. Originally indigenous to Jamaica, JVS has been reported in the United States and other parts of the world, possibly due to canned ackee fruit imported from Jamaica. The ackee plant was named one of the world's most dangerous foods by *Travel + Leisure* magazine.

Korsakoff Syndrome: a chronic memory disorder caused by a lack of Thiamine (Vitamin B-1) in the brain. Symptoms are amnesia, lack of coordination, confabulation, and disorientation. Alcoholism is often the cause of this condition, though it may also be associated with malnutrition, eating disorders, chronic infections, AIDS, or other illnesses. Korsakoff may also be referred to as amnesiac syndrome, and is sometimes related to Wernicke's encephalopathy.

Lactose Intolerance: inability to digest lactose which causes bloating, cramps, diarrhea, gas, and nausea. *Olympic swimmer Mark Spitz, music producer Randy Jackson, actress/comedian Whoopi Goldberg, actress Lisa Kudrow, TV personality Star Jones, boxer Oscar de la Hoya, actor/comedian John Cleese.*

Lupus: a chronic, inflammatory, autoimmune disease also referred to as systemic lupus erythematosus (SLE). As with many of the mystery diseases, lupus is of unknown origin, difficult to diagnose, and has no cure. *Singer Toni Braxton, baseball star Tim Raines, singer Seal, journalist Charles Kuralt.*

Lyme Disease (Borreliosis): a disease caused by the bacterium Borrelia Burgdorferi which can be transmitted to humans via the bite of a deer tick. Even with a raised level of awareness about Lyme, it remains a mystifying and hard-to-diagnose disease. If caught early, Lyme disease can usually be cured; but its symptoms are vague and often mimic those of other illnesses, making it difficult to diagnose. In addition, blood tests for Lyme often give false results, especially early on in the progression of the illness. If Lyme progresses unchecked for more than a year, the effects can be devastating.

Author Amy Tan, singer Daryl Hall, actor Parker Posey, President George W. Bush.

Mad Cow Disease: a progressive neurological disorder of cattle that is sometimes transmitted to humans who consume contaminated beef. Mad Cow is also known as Bovine Spongiform Encephalopathy (BSE) and appears to be related to Creutzfeldt-Jakob Disease (CJD).

Meniere's Disease: a chronic vestibular disorder in which excess fluid in the inner ear causes vertigo, dizziness, tinnitus, headache, hearing loss, gastrointestinal disturbances, and other symptoms. There is no known cause or cure.

Singer Ryan Adams, pianist/composer David Alstead, astronaut Alan Shepard, author Jonathan Swift, guitarist Les Paul.

MERS-CoV: a deadly, new SARS-like virus (called the novel coronavirus) identified in May, 2013. It can cause severe fever, cough, respiratory problems, diarrhea, pneumonia, and kidney failure. At this time, very little is known about this disease except that half of those afflicted with MERS-CoV will die.

Migraine: extremely painful headache that can often be accompanied by nausea, vomiting, ringing in the ears, dizziness, seeing zigzag lines, blind spots, and extreme sensitivity to light.

Tennis star Serena Williams, actor Ben Affleck, actress Lisa Kudrow, singer Janet Jackson, Congresswoman Michele Bachmann, football star Troy Aikman.

Morgellons Disease: one of the more controversial and least understood disorders. People with Morgellons have the feeling that bugs are crawling on them or that tiny fibers are stuck in their skin. They also complain of sores, burning, stinging and intense itching of the skin. The medical community is divided regarding Morgellons. Some call it an unexplained dermopathy, a skin condition that occurs without a known reason. Others categorize it as a type of psychosis known as delusional parasitosis, in which a person believes that parasites have invaded their skin. Others suggest it is a disease caused by genetically modified foods or by pesticides.
Singer Joni Mitchell, baseball player Billy Koch.

Multiple Sclerosis (MS): an autoimmune disease that affects the brain, spinal cord, and entire central nervous system. Like many of the mystery diseases, MS is of unknown origin and causes a wide range of disturbing symptoms, including weakness, numbness, vision loss, tremors, slurred speech, and fatigue.
Television personality Montel Williams, actress Teri Garr, news anchor Neil Cavuto, journalist Richard Cohen, actress Annette Funicello, comedian/actor Richard Pryor.

Mysophobia (Germophobia): an irrational, obsessive and exaggerated fear of germs.
Actor/comedian Howie Mandel, actress Cameron Diaz, TV/radio host Glenn Beck, actress/model Megan Fox.

Narcolepsy: extreme daytime sleepiness that can cause sufferers to fall asleep suddenly, even during activities such as talking or eating.
Television personality Jimmy Kimmel, abolitionist Harriet Tubman, Professor George M. Church, politician Harold Ickes.

Obsessive Compulsive Disorder (OCD): an anxiety disorder characterized by unreasonable and unwanted thoughts and fears. The sufferer performs repetitive or ritualistic behaviors in an effort to ease their distress and anxiety.

Actress Jessica Alba, actress Charlize Theron, minister Martin Luther, inventor Nikola Tesla, Confederate General Stonewall Jackson, actor Leonardo Dicaprio, businessman Howard Hughes.

Other Specified Feeding and Eating Disorders (OSFED): eating disorder category for patients who meet some, but not all, of the criteria for bulimia or anorexia. Symptoms may include chewing and spitting out large amounts of food, or forcing oneself to vomit after eating normal food amounts. (*see EDNOS.) According to a 2012 study in the *International Journal of Eating Disorders*, eating disorders now affect 13% of American women age 50 or older. Once considered mainly a problem for teenagers and young adults, life-threatening eating disorders are now increasing at a disturbing rate in older Americans.

Pancreatitis: inflammation of the pancreas, the large gland behind the stomach that releases digestive enzymes into the small intestine, and releases insulin and glucagon into the bloodstream. Bile duct stones or heavy alcohol use can cause pancreatitis, but in some cases the cause is not known. The number of cases of pancreatitis has risen sharply since the 1980's; nearly a quarter of a million people are hospitalized each year, and there are nearly 2500 deaths.

Composer Ludwig von Beethoven, jazz musician Dizzie Gillepsie, Macedonian King Alexander the Great, actor Matthew Perry.

Panic Disorder (PD): an anxiety disorder characterized by repeated attacks of intense fear that trigger severe physical reactions when there is no real danger or apparent cause.
Baseball star Joey Votto, actor Johnny Depp, singer Adele, inventor Nikola Tesla, singer Carrie Underwood.

Parkinson's Disease: a progressive disorder of the nervous system that causes tremor, slowed movements, rigid muscles, speech difficulties, and other symptoms. The cause and cure are unknown.
Boxer Muhammad Ali, actor Michael J. Fox, actor James Doohan, U.S. Attorney General Janet Reno, Reverend Billy Graham, singer Johnny Cash, cartoonist Charles Schulz.

Persistent Genital Arousal Disorder (PGAD): unwanted spontaneous and unrelenting genital arousal in women that occurs without sexual stimulation. May be grouped with priapism (persistent penile erection) in men.

Pica Disorder: an insatiable, persistent desire to eat dirt, paint, or other non-food substances. There is no known cause or cure.

Prosopagnosia (Face Blindness): An impairment in the recognition of faces. Prosopagnosics often have difficulty recognizing family members, close friends, and even themselves. Other types of recognition impairments (place, car, facial expression of emotion) often accompany this condition.
Actor Brad Pitt, neurologist Oliver Sacks, painter Chuck Close.

Prostatitis, Chronic: an inflammation, often of unknown origin, of the prostate gland that can cause general bodily pain (particularly in the perineum area), fatigue, sexual dysfunction, and pain during urination and ejaculation. Chronic prostatitis is a painful, troubling condition that affects nearly two million American men, comes and goes over time, and may or may not be related to a bacterial infection. The website prostatitis.org makes this disturbing statement: "The current state of scientific and medical knowledge about prostatitis is not very good." Surprising new research indicates that this distressing condition may not be related to the prostate gland at all, but may rather be an autoimmune ailment better known as Chronic Pelvic Pain Syndrome (CPPS).

Q Fever: a bacterial infection that causes flu-like symptoms for several weeks, and can also seriously damage various parts of the body including the heart, lungs, and liver. It is caused by the resilient bacteria *Coxiella burnetii* which infects dogs, cats, sheep, goats, and many other animals. Humans can contract Q Fever by breathing in contaminated droplets released by infected animals. The "Q" stands for "Query" because researchers who originally studied the mysterious disease in 1937 had more questions than answers. The largest known outbreak of Q Fever affected 4000 humans in the Netherlands from 2007-2010.

Raynaud's Disease: condition which causes blood vessel spasms that block blood flow to hands, feet, fingers, toes, ears and nose. May be precipitated by cold temperatures or strong emotions, but there is often no apparent precursor. This disorder causes extreme numbness, pain, cold and drastic changes in the color of the skin.

Reiter's Syndrome: a form of arthritis that causes inflammation of the joints, eyes, and urinary, genital, or

gastrointestinal tract. Also known as reactive arthritis and is one of the spondyloarthropathy disorders.
Explorer Christopher Columbus.

Restless Leg Syndrome (RLS): neurological movement disorder that interrupts sleep and causes extreme discomfort in the legs and an overwhelming urge to move them. Also known as Willis-Ekbom Disease.
Actor Taylor Lautner, TV personality Keith Olbermann.

Rheumatoid Arthritis (RA): an inflammatory arthritis and autoimmune disease of unknown origin. The body's immune system attacks the lining of the joints causing pain and inflammation throughout the body.
Actress Kathleen Turner, French impressionist painter Pierre-Auguste Renoir, x-ray pioneer/Nobel prize winner Dorothy Hodgkin, actor James Coburn, Dr. Christiann Barnard.

Sarcoid: an inflammatory disease that affects multiple organs in the body, but mostly the lungs and lymph nodes.
Entertainer Bernie Mac, professional football star Reggie White.

Schizophrenia: A chronic, severe brain disorder that interrupts a person's ability to accurately perceive the world and process information. Symptoms may include poor concentration, memory loss, lack of emotion, hallucinations, delusions, and many others.
Mathematician/Nobel prize winner John Forbes Nash, rock musician Syd Barrett, jazz musician Tom Harrell, first lady Mary Todd Lincoln, author Jack Kerouac.

Scleroderma: a chronic connective tissue disease generally regarded as autoimmune rheumatic in nature.

171

This dangerous disease hardens skin tissues, damages internal organs, and constricts blood flow.

Self-harm or self-mutilation: a psychological disorder that causes one to inflict intentional injury to one's own body. Includes burning, excessive piercing, cutting, hitting, and head-banging.
Singer Fiona Apple, comedian/actor Russell Brand, English athlete Kelly Holmes, author/researcher Alfred Kinsey, actress Demi Lovato, Olympic swimmer Amanda Beard.

Severe Acute Respiratory Syndrome (SARS): a deadly respiratory disease that typically attacks the lungs but may also affect the gastrointestinal tract. SARS is a member of the coronavirus family of viruses (the same as that which causes the common cold) and was first identified in 2003.

Shingles (Herpes Zoster): typically appears as a very painful skin rash on the torso or face, although some people have very little or no rash at all. A variety of other symptoms may also accompany the rash, and can continue off and on for weeks, months or years. Shingles is caused by the varicella-zoster virus, the same one which causes chicken pox. After a person contracts chicken pox, the virus remains dormant for years in various nerve roots; and for some unknown reason, reactivates later in life to cause shingles. Formerly a disease confined almost entirely to the elderly, shingles is now markedly on the rise in younger age groups. The reason is not known.
Former President Richard Nixon, baseball manager Tony LaRussa, actor Frank Langella, former Israeli Prime Minister Golda Meir, singer Amy Grant.

Sjogren's Syndrome: this inflammatory disease and chronic disorder of the immune system causes a variety of arthritic symptoms and attacks the body's glands, particularly those that lubricate the eyes, ears, and nose.
Tennis star Venus Williams.

Sleep Apnea: a serious sleep disorder in which breathing is interrupted repeatedly during sleep.
Basketball star Shaquille O'Neal, singer/musician Jerry Garcia, comedian/TV personality Rosie O'Donnell, TV personality Regis Philbin.

Social Anxiety Disorder (SAD): a disorder in which common, normal social interactions or settings cause extreme, irrational fear, embarrassment, and anxiety. Also known as Social Phobia.
Football star Ricky Williams, actress Kim Basinger, baseball star Zach Greinke, singer/actor Donny Osmond, singer Barbara Streisand.

Synesthesia: a disorder in which one type of sensory stimulation evokes a different sort of sensory response. For example, hearing the sound of a bell might produce the image of the color blue in a person's mind. Or seeing a candle might elicit the taste of a glazed doughnut. For some with synesthesia, the condition is a pleasant and useful facet of their lives, but for others it can be a serious distraction in business meetings, while reading or driving, or in other daily activities.
Russian composer Nikolai Rimsky-Korskov, artist David Hockney, rapper Pharrell Williams, author Vladimir Nabokov, jazz composer Duke Ellington.

Thoracic Outlet Syndrome (TOS): compression of the nerves, arteries and veins in the lower neck and upper chest area which causes pain in the arms, shoulders and neck. This condition may present symptoms similar to fibromyalgia, multiple sclerosis, and complex regional pain syndrome, and is difficult to diagnose or treat. TOS may be caused by many things, from stress to tumors to playing sports like baseball and volleyball.

Professional baseball players Hank Blalock, Matt Harrison, Jeremy Bonderman, Chris Carpenter.

Tinnitus: a common problem that affects about 20% of the population. Tinnitus is described as a noise or ringing sound in the ears, and is widely considered to be a symptom of an underlying issue such as aging, ear damage, or a circulatory disorder. Tinnitus is not considered a serious ailment, but can be very distressing and life-affecting when the ringing, buzzing, whistling and clicking noises continue at a very loud level for days at a time.

Television personality William Shatner, singer Barbara Streisand, actor Sylvester Stallone, inventor Thomas Edison, talk show host David Letterman.

Tourette's Disorder: a brain condition that typically begins in childhood, and causes a person to perform repetitive sounds or movements (tics) that they can't control.

Businessman/billionaire Howard Hughes, soccer player Tim Howard, auto racer Steve Wallace, baseball player Jim Eisenreich.

Transient Global Amnesia (TGA): a sudden, temporary loss of memory that is not attributed to a neurological condition such as stroke or epilepsy. TGA can be caused by a variety of things including acute emotional distress, sudden immersion in cold or hot water, sexual intercourse or other strenuous physical activity. This condition typically resolves within 24 hours.

Trichotillomania: a mysterious, complex, psychological disorder in which the sufferer has the irresistible urge to pull out his own hair.
Actress/model Olivia Munn.

Uncombable Hair Syndrome (UHS): a rare condition that affects the hair shafts of the scalp. Hair progressively becomes straw-like, dry and disordered, sticking straight out from the head, and almost impossible to manage. UHS is often a genetic disorder but may also occur spontaneously. It may sometimes also be referred to as "spun glass hair."

Usher Syndrome: rare disease that affects both hearing and vision, and causes hearing loss, deafness, night blindness and tunnel vision.
Singer Rigoberto Tovar Garcia.

Vulvar Vestibulitis Syndrome (Vulvodynia): a condition of unexplained vulvar pain for women that can cause physical disabilities, limitation of activities, sexual dysfunction, and psychological distress. This condition has been steadily on the rise in recent decades, but is often misdiagnosed or even downplayed by some physicians. The cause of vulvodynia is unknown and is rarely remedied with existing therapies or medications.

Waldmann Disease: a digestive disorder characterized by enlarged lymph vessels in the lining of the small intestine. This condition causes a leaking of lymphatic fluid and protein into the gastrointestinal tract, fewer antibodies in the blood, and immunodeficiency. The cause of Waldmann Disease is unknown, and it is often fatal.

Watermelon Stomach (WMS): a condition in which the lining of the stomach bleeds, giving it the appearance (when viewed during endoscopy) like the lines on the outside of a watermelon. This disorder causes sudden, unexplained bleeding, vomiting of blood, blood in stool, and anemia. The cause of Watermelon Stomach is unknown and there is no cure.

Werewolf Diseases (Hypertrichosis): very rare condition with fewer than 100 documented cases that causes a person to grow thick groupings of hair on various parts of the face and body. It may manifest as generalized (hair all over the body) or localized (hair only on specific parts of the body). Some cases of Hypertrichosis are caused by a genetic mutation on the X chromosome, but others are acquired later in life, possibly due to drug use, eating disorders, or cancer. There is currently no cure.
Jo-Jo the Dog-Faced Boy (Barnum & Bailey Circus), Supatra "Nat" Sasuphan (the world's hairiest child).

Zygomycosis (Mucormycosis): a fungal infection that occurs most often in the sinuses, brain, or lungs; but it may also be found in the gastrointestinal tract, liver, or on the skin. It is caused by a common fungus found in the soil or in dying plants. Zygomycosis usually strikes people with a weakened immune system (though not always), and is often fatal, even with aggressive treatment. This infection was responsible for the deaths of at least three survivors of the tornado in Joplin, Missouri, in 2011.

7517425R00099

Printed in Great Britain
by Amazon.co.uk, Ltd.,
Marston Gate.